PLANT BASED COOKBOOK FOR BEGINNERS
2024:

EXPLORING YOUR GUIDE TO WHOLESOME DELICIOUS AND HEALTHY VEGAN MEALS WHILE BEING CREATIVE.

BY

CODY LOWE

Introduction

CHAPTER ONE

How come plant based foods?

Benefits of plant-based diets

Is a plant-based diet for you?

CHAPTER TWO

BREAKFAST

VEGAN PANCAKE

ACAI BOWL

SPINACH AND MUSHROOM VEGAN OMELETTE

VEGAN BANANA BREAD

CHIA SEEDS PUDDING WITH BERRIES

VEGAN TOFU SCRAMBLE

OATMEAL WITH ALMOND BUTTER AND BANANA

AVOCADO TOAST WITH CHICKPEAS

QUINOA BREAKFAST BOWL

VEGAN BREAKFAST SANDWICH

AVOCADO AND TOMATO TOAST

VEGAN BREAKFAST BURRITO

SWEET POTATO AND KALE HASH

CINNAMON APPLE OVERNIGHT OATS

SMOOTHIE BOWL

PUMPKIN SPICE CHIA PUDDING

VEGAN WAFFLES

VEGAN FRENCH TOAST

SAUTÉED SPINACH AND MUSHROOM BAGEL

CAULIFLOWER BREAKFAST BURRITOS

CHAPTER THREE

LUNCH

VEGAN MINESTRONE SOUP

VEGAN EGGPLANT PARMESAN

TOMATO BASIL QUINOA BOWL

VEGAN GREEK SALAD WRAP

LENTIL SOUP

VEGAN MEDITERRANEAN PIZZA

SPAGHETTI AGLIO E OLIO WITH BROCCOLI

CAPRESE SALAD WITH VEGAN MOZZARELLA

VEGAN SUSHI ROLLS

PESTO ZOODLES

STIR-FRIED TOFU AND VEGGIES

CAULIFLOWER BUFFALO WINGS SALAD

VEGAN BBQ JACKFRUIT SANDWICH

THAI COCONUT CURRY SOUP

CREAMY BROCCOLI AND POTATO SOUP

PUMPKIN AND LENTIL CURRY

SWEET POTATO AND BLACK BEAN QUESADILLA

MEXICAN QUINOA SALAD

VEGAN BLT SANDWICH

CHICKPEA AND SPINACH CURRY

CHAPTER FOUR

DINNER

VEGAN SPAGHETTI BOLOGNESE
LEMON HERB QUINOA SALAD
VEGAN BUDDHA BOWL
VEGAN SPINACH AND ARTICHOKE
VEGAN TERIYAKI TEMPEH BOWL
VEGAN GNOCCHI WITH TOMATO BASIL SAUCE
VEGAN STUFFED MUSHROOM
VEGAN PHO
QUINOA STUFFED BELL PEPPER
VEGAN PAD THAI
CHICKPEA AND SPINACH STEW
VEGAN SHEPHERD'S PIE
VEGAN LENTIL LOAF
VEGAN STUFFED ACORN SQUASH
PLANT-BASED LASAGNA
CHICKPEA STIR-FRY WITH BROCCOLI
VEGAN LENTIL TACOS
VEGAN RATATOUILLE
MUSHROOM RISOTTO
VEGAN BURRITO BOWL
CHAPTER FIVE
DELICIOUS DESSERTS
ALMOND BUTTER ENERGY BALLS
MATCHA GREEN TEA ICE CREAM
VEGAN CHOCOLATE AVOCADO COOKIES
VEGAN TIRAMISU
VEGAN CHOCOLATE CAKE
CHOCOLATE AVOCADO PUDDING

VEGAN APPLE CRISP
NO-BAKE VEGAN CHEESECAKE BITES
COCONUT MANGO SORBET
VEGAN BANANA BREAD
PISTACHIO DATES BITES
VEGAN CINNAMON ROLLS
RASPBERRY ALMOND THUMBPRINT
COOKIES
STRAWBERRY BANANA NICE CREAM
CHOCOLATE DIPPED STRAWBERRIES
AVOCADO CHOCOLATE MOUSSE
VEGAN BLUEBERRY CHEESECAKES
VEGAN LEMON BARS
PEANUT BUTTER OAT COOKIES
PUMPKIN SPICE ENERGY BITES
Conclusion

Introduction

Welcome to the exciting world of plant-based eating, where flavor, sustainability, and health join together to completely transform your experience with food. This thorough book is designed with novices in mind, acting as a road map for navigating the vast array of plant-based cooking options. You'll discover the delight of cooking tasty, filling meals as well as the nutritional advantages as you set out on this life-changing journey. We urge you to discover the art of plant-based cooking and discover a world of flavors that nourish the body and the soul, from simple and quick recipes to creative creations.

Eating plant-based is not only delicious and full of gourmet experiences, but it also has many health advantages. Rich in antioxidants, vitamins, and minerals, plant-based meals promote general health. They frequently have reduced cholesterol and saturated fat contents, which supports heart health and lowers the chance of developing chronic illnesses. You're providing your body with healthy, nutrient-dense foods as you enjoy the tastes of your plant-based recipes.

Make sure you have fun on this adventure!

CHAPTER ONE

How come plant based foods?

Plant-based diets have a long and rich history that is entwined with philosophical, religious, and cultural beliefs. Plant-based eating has gained popularity in the modern era, but its development has been shaped by historical movements and practices.

Ancient Civilizations:

- A large number of ancient civilizations, such as Greece and Rome, relied largely on grains, vegetables, and legumes in their plant-based diets.

- Vegetarianism has roots in religious and philosophical traditions such as Jainism and Hinduism in some Eastern cultures, like India. Religious and Philosophical Influences: Dietary practices were frequently influenced by religious beliefs. For instance, plant-based diets were encouraged in some Christian monastic traditions.

- Principles of Buddhism and Jainism emphasize compassion and non-harm towards all living things, which supports plant-based and vegetarian diets.

Early Vegetarian Movements:

- Vegetarian movements became popular in North America and Europe during the 1800s. Plant-based diets were encouraged by proponents like Sylvester Graham and John Harvey Kellogg for health-related reasons. The Vegetarian Society was instrumental

in bringing vegetarianism to a wider audience. It was established in the United Kingdom in 1847.
The twentieth century and veganism: One of The Vegan Society's founders, Donald Watson, first used the term "vegan" in 1944. Beyond just eating a plant-based diet, veganism involves giving up all animal products, such as dairy and eggs. In the second half of the 20th century, plant-based and vegan diets gained popularity due to ethical and environmental concerns.
Health Movements and Scientific Support: - As scientific research on the advantages of plant-based diets became more widely available in the late 20th and early 21st centuries, public interest in these dietary practices grew.
  - The acceptance of plant-based eating was further enhanced by organizations such as the American Dietetic Association, which recognized well-planned vegetarian diets as appropriate for all life stages.
The current surge in popularity: Plant-based diets have gained significant popularity in recent decades due to ethical, environmental, and health-related factors.
  - The mainstreaming of plant-based eating can be attributed to celebrities, documentaries, and significant individuals. Terms like "flexitarian," "plant-based," and "vegan" are becoming more commonly used.

Benefits of plant-based diets

Diets based mostly on plants have many health advantages. Because of their high fiber, vitamin, and antioxidant content, they help to maintain digestive health and lower the risk of developing chronic illnesses like heart disease and some types of cancer. These diets frequently result in improved blood pressure management and decreased cholesterol. Plant-based diets also aid in weight management because they typically contain fewer calories and saturated fats.
Eating a plant-based diet benefits the environment in addition to one's own health. Compared to animal agriculture, it uses less land, water, and resources, which helps to reduce greenhouse gas emissions and environmental degradation. This environmentally friendly feature supports sustainable objectives. In general, adopting a plant-based diet can improve sustainability of the environment as well as personal well-being.

Is a plant-based diet for you?

Choosing to adopt a plant-based diet is a personal decision that is impacted by environmental awareness, ethical convictions, and health goals. Investigating plant-based recipes is often the first step toward better health and a stronger bond with the environment.
Health Considerations: There are numerous health advantages to a plant-based diet high in fruits, vegetables, whole grains, and legumes. Such diets

may help improve weight control, heart health, and lower the risk of chronic diseases, according to research. Novices frequently find the shift to be gradual, enjoying the higher intake of antioxidants, fiber, and vitamins found in plant-based foods. Impact on the Environment and Animal Welfare: Ethical considerations for plant-based diets go beyond health issues to include issues of environmental sustainability and animal welfare. Selecting plant-based alternatives is in line with compassion principles because it lessens the environmental impact of meat production and decreases dependency on animal products. Plant-based recipes provide a practical means of making good decisions on a daily basis for individuals who are driven by ethical and environmental concerns.

Making the Transition: Beginner-friendly plant-based recipes offer a welcome introduction to this dietary change. The wide range of tastes, textures, and cooking options guarantees that the shift is both enjoyable and health-conscious while also encouraging the discovery of new flavors. The learning curve is made fun by easy substitutions, inventive combinations, and the use of herbs and spices, which inspires people to explore the culinary artistry of plant-based cuisine. A plant-based diet may or may not be the best option for you, depending on your particular values, health goals, and personal preferences. If you plan to make big dietary changes, it's best to speak with a medical practitioner or a registered dietitian. The transition to a plant-based diet is an exciting and fulfilling one that can lead to better health as well as a meaningful contribution to a world that is more sustainable and compassionate.

<u>CHAPTER TWO</u>

BREAKFAST

VEGAN PANCAKE

Ingredients: - One cup of whole wheat or all-purpose flour - One tablespoon of sugar - Two teaspoons of baking powder
- 1 cup plant-based milk (oat, soy, or almond milk work well) - 1/8 teaspoon salt
- Melted coconut oil or two tablespoons of vegetable oil - One teaspoon of vanilla extract

Guidelines:
1. Combine the flour, sugar, baking powder, and salt in a sizable mixing bowl.
2. Combine the plant-based milk, vegetable oil, and vanilla essence in another bowl.
3. Add the wet mixture to the dry mixture and whisk just until blended. A few lumps are acceptable because overmixing can cause the pancakes to become dense.
4. Turn up the heat to medium in a nonstick skillet or griddle. Apply a thin layer of cooking spray or oil to the surface.
5. For each pancake, pour 1/4 cup of batter into the skillet. Cook until the edges start to look set and bubbles appear on the surface.

6. After flipping, fry the pancake till golden brown on the opposite side. Usually, each side takes one to two minutes to complete.
7. Continue until all of the batter has been used, reducing the heat as needed to avoid burning.
8. Top the warm pancakes with your preferred toppings, including fresh fruit, maple syrup, or a dollop of vegan yogurt.

Cooking Time: - Pancakes normally take 1-2 minutes to cook on each side, therefore the total amount of time needed to prepare a batch of pancakes is about 4/6 minutes.

ACAI BOWL

Ingredients:
 - Two packs of frozen, unsweetened ACAI puree Plant-based milk (coconut, soy, or almond): 1/2 to 1 cup
- One sliced ripe banana
- Half a cup of frozen berry mixture
– One to two teaspoons of nut butter (almond or peanut).
- Additions of granola, sliced strawberries, chia seeds, coconut flakes, and extra banana slices

Guidelines
1. Split the Acai Packs
 To gently thaw, run some warm water over the frozen Acai packets for a few seconds. Cut them up into pieces.

2. Combine other ingredients with acai.

Place the frozen berries, banana slices, nut butter, plant-based milk, and Acai bits in a blender. Puree until a thick, creamy consistency is reached. It might be necessary to pause and scrape down the edges to make sure everything is thoroughly mixed.

3. Modify Uniformity

If more plant-based milk is required to get the right thickness, add it.

4. Get the toppings ready.

Cut bananas and strawberries into slices. Collect additional garnishes such as chia seeds, coconut flakes, and granola.

5. Place Acai Bowl together.

Transfer the mixed Acai blend into a bowl.

6. Include toppings

Top with banana slices, granola, coconut flakes, chia seeds, and sliced strawberries.

7. Present Right Away

The optimum time to eat acai bowls is right away, while they're still chilly and cool.

SPINACH AND MUSHROOM VEGAN OMELETTE

Ingredients:

1 cup besan, or chickpea flour (sometimes called gram flour).

– 1 tablespoon nutritional yeast

– 1 1/4 cups water

- Half a teaspoon of powdered sugar

- One-half teaspoon of powdered turmeric
- One tablespoon of olive oil
- Salt and pepper to taste
- One cup chopped fresh spinach
 - One cup sliced mushrooms
- 1/4 cup sliced red bell pepper (optional)
One quarter cup of finely chopped onion (optional)
- Vegan cheese (as an optional filler)

Guidelines:

To make the batter, combine the chickpea flour, water, nutritional yeast, baking powder, turmeric powder, salt, and pepper in a mixing bowl. Verify that there are no lumps.

2. Sauté Vegetables: - In a nonstick skillet set over medium heat, heat the olive oil.

   Incorporate finely chopped spinach, red bell pepper, onion, and mushrooms, if desired. Vegetables should be sautéed till soft.

3. Add Batter: - Evenly cover the sautéed veggies with the chickpea flour batter.

4. Cook Omelet: - Cook until the bottom is golden brown and the edges begin to firm, a few minutes. To aid with the top cook, you can place a lid on the skillet.

5. Optional Filling: - You can top one half of the omelette with vegan cheese if you'd like.

6. Fold and Serve: - Using a spatula, gently fold the omelette in half once it has set mostly.

   - Cook the omelette for one more minute, or until it is thoroughly done.

7. Serve Warm: Transfer the plant-based omelette to a platter and proceed to serve it warm.
Cooking Time: Depending on the heat settings on your stove, the vegan omelette will take about 10 to 15 minutes to cook in total. The key is to ensure that the omelette is cooked through and has a golden-brown color on both sides.

VEGAN BANANA BREAD

Ingredients:
 - 3 mashed ripe bananas
- 1 teaspoon vanilla extract - 1/2 cup agave nectar or maple syrup - 1/3 cup melted coconut oil or vegetable oil
One and a quarter cups all-purpose flour; one tsp baking soda
- 1/4 teaspoon salt - 1/2 teaspoon (optional) ground cinnamon
- 1/2 cup of chocolate chips or chopped nuts (optional)

Guidelines:
1. Preheat Oven: Set the oven's temperature to 350°F, or 175°C. Grease a 9x5-inch loaf pan.
2. Mash Bananas: Use a fork or potato masher to mash the ripe bananas in a large mixing bowl.
3. Add Wet Ingredients: - To the mashed bananas, add vanilla extract, melted coconut oil or vegetable oil, and maple syrup or agave nectar. Blend thoroughly.

4. Combine Dry Ingredients: - Beat flour, baking soda, salt, and ground cinnamon (if using) in a separate bowl.

5. Mix the Wet and Dry Ingredients: - Gently stir the dry ingredients into the wet ingredients after adding them. Be careful not to over mix.

6. Optional Add-ins: - If preferred, mix chocolate chips or chopped nuts into the batter.

7. Pour into Pan: - Fill the loaf pan with batter after it has been greased.

8. Bake: - Bake for 60–70 minutes, or until a toothpick inserted in the center comes out clean, or with a few moist crumbs, depending on the oven.

9. Cool: After letting the banana bread cool in the pan for roughly ten minutes, move it to a wire rack to finish cooling.

Cooking Time:

- The baking time for vegan banana bread is approximately 60-70 minutes at 350°F (175°C). Keep an eye on it, as actual cooking times may vary based on your oven.

CHIA SEEDS PUDDING WITH BERRIES

Ingredients:
- 1/4 cup chia seeds
- 1 cup plant-based milk (almond, coconut, or soy)
- 1-2 tablespoons (adjust to taste) of agave or maple syrup
- 1/2 teaspoon vanilla extract

- Mixed berries (strawberries, blueberries, raspberries) for topping

Guidelines:
1. Combine Chia Seeds with Liquid: - Place chia seeds, plant-based milk, maple syrup, and vanilla extract in a bowl or jar.
2. Stir Well: - Make sure the chia seeds are dispersed evenly and do not clump together by giving the mixture a good stir.
3. Chill: - Place a lid on the bowl or jar and place it in the fridge for a minimum of three hours, or better yet, overnight. This enables the liquid to be absorbed by the chia seeds, giving the mixture a pudding-like consistency.
4. Stir Once More: - Give the chia pudding another stir following the first refrigeration period. To get the right consistency, thin it out with a little more plant-based milk if it's too thick.
5. Present with Berries: - Ladle the pudding made with chia seeds into bowls or jars for serving.
   - Add a heaping helping of mixed berries on top.
6. Optional Add-ons: If you'd like, feel free to add more toppings like chopped nuts, sliced bananas, or a drizzle of nut butter.

Chia seed pudding is a healthy and adaptable breakfast option. Savor the berries' creamy texture and crisp burst of freshness!

VEGAN TOFU SCRAMBLE

Ingredients:
- 1 block (about 14-16 oz) firm tofu, pressed and crumbled
- 1 tablespoon olive oil
- 1 small onion, diced
- 1 bell pepper, diced
- 2 cloves garlic, minced
- 1 teaspoon turmeric powder (for color)
- 1/2 teaspoon cumin
- 1/2 teaspoon paprika
- Salt and pepper to taste
- Optional: Spinach, tomatoes, nutritional yeast, or black salt for added flavor

Guidelines:
1. Tofu preparation:
Squeeze out any excess water by pressing the tofu. You have two options: use a tofu press for 15 to 30 minutes, or cover the tofu block with a clean kitchen towel and something heavy.After being pressed, use your hands to crumble the tofu.
2. Sauté Vegetables:
 - Heat the olive oil in a large skillet over medium heat. Add the chopped onion and bell pepper. vegetables should be sautéed until they are soft.
3. Include the tofu and spices:
Add the crumbled tofu to the skillet. Add the paprika, turmeric powder, cumin, salt, and pepper along with the minced garlic. To evenly distribute the spices, give it a good stir.

4. Cook and Stir:
 - Cook, stirring frequently, for about 8 to 10 minutes with the tofu mixture. This gives the tofu a slightly crispy texture and allows it to absorb the flavors.
5. Optional Add-ins:
- Include extras like tomatoes or spinach. Stir until thoroughly heated or wilted.
6. Modify Seasoning:
- Taste the tofu scramble and make any required adjustments to the seasoning. For an eggy taste, you can add a small pinch of black salt.
7. Serve Warm:
– After the tofu is done to your satisfaction, proceed to serve the scramble hot.

Cooking Time: - The vegan tofu scramble takes about 15 to 20 minutes to prepare in total. It's important to cook the tofu until it acquires the right texture and absorbs the flavors of the veggies and spices.

OATMEAL WITH ALMOND BUTTER AND BANANA

Ingredients:
- 1 cup rolled oats
- 2 cups plant-based milk (almond, soy, or oat milk)
- 1 ripe banana, mashed
- 2 tablespoons almond butter
- Optional toppings: Sliced banana, chopped nuts, a drizzle of maple syrup

Guidelines:

1. Cook Oats:

- Put plant-based milk and rolled oats in a saucepan.

2. Bring to a Simmer:

 - Over medium heat, bring the mixture to a simmer, stirring from time to time.

3. Mash Banana: Mash the ripe banana in a bowl while the oats are cooking.

4. Add Banana to Oats:

- Stir in the mashed banana once the oats have absorbed the majority of the liquid and reached the desired consistency.

5. Add Almond Butter and Stir Well:

- Add almond butter to the oatmeal and stir well.

6. Cook to the Correct Consistency:

 Cook the oatmeal for a few more minutes or until the desired thickness is achieved. You can thin it out with additional plant-based milk if necessary.

7. Serve Warm:

- After the oatmeal is cooked to your preference, take it off the stove and give it a minute to rest. Next, serve it hot.

8. Top as Desired:

 - If you'd like, top the oatmeal with chopped nuts, sliced bananas, or a drizzle of maple syrup.

Cooking Time: Depending on the type of oats used and the desired thickness, oatmeal typically takes 5 to 10 minutes to cook through. Observe the consistency and modify the cooking time as necessary.

AVOCADO TOAST WITH CHICKPEAS

Ingredients:
- 2 slices of whole-grain bread
- 1 ripe avocado
- scoop out and rinse one cup of canned chickpeas
- 1 tablespoon olive oil
- 1 teaspoon smoked paprika
- Salt and pepper to taste
- Optional toppings: Red pepper flakes, lemon juice, microgreens

Guidelines:
1. Toast the Bread:
 - Toast the whole-grain bread slices until they are to your preference.
2. Prepare the avocado:
 Cut the ripe avocado in half, take out the pit, and scoop out the flesh into a bowl while the bread is toasting. Using a fork, mash it and add salt and pepper to taste.
3. Sauté the chickpeas:
- Heat the olive oil in a skillet over medium heat. until they are thoroughly heated and spiced.
4. Assemble Avocado Toast:
 - Evenly spread each slice of toasted bread with mashed avocado.
5. Add Chickpeas on Top:

- Place a spoonful of the sautéed chickpeas over the avocado mash.
6. Add Optional Toppings:
- To add some freshness, you can optionally drizzle some lemon juice, add some red pepper flakes, and top with microgreens.
7. Serve Right Away:
- While the avocado toast and chickpeas are still warm, serve them right away.

Cooking Time: - It takes a few minutes to toast the bread and roughly five minutes to sauté the chickpeas. About ten minutes should pass during the entire process.

QUINOA BREAKFAST BOWL

Ingredients:
- 1 cup quinoa, rinsed
- 2 cups plant-based milk (almond, soy, or oat milk)
1/4 cup agave nectar or maple syrup
- 1/2 teaspoon vanilla extract
- Toppings: Fresh berries, sliced banana, nuts, seeds, or dried fruits

Guidelines:
1. Rinse Quinoa:
To get rid of any bitterness, rinse the quinoa under cold water.
2. Prepare the Quinoa:
 - Place the rinsed quinoa, plant-based milk, maple syrup, and vanilla extract in a saucepan.
3. Bring to a Boil:

Using medium-high heat, bring the mixture to a boil.
4. Simmer:
- Lower the heat to a simmer, place a lid on the saucepan, and allow the quinoa to cook and absorb the liquid for 15 to 20 minutes.
5. Fluff Quinoa: Use a fork to fluff the cooked quinoa.
6. Add Toppings:
 - Sprinkle dried fruits, nuts, seeds, or sliced bananas on top of each bowl.
8. Optional Sweeten Even More:
 - If you'd like, pour a little bit more agave nectar or maple syrup on top for sweetness.

Cooking Time: Quinoa takes about 15 to 20 minutes to cook through. Remember that quinoa is done when the grains are soft and the liquid has been absorbed.

VEGAN BREAKFAST SANDWICH

Ingredients:
- 1 block of firm tofu, sliced and pressed into slabs that are 1/2 inch thick.
- 2 tablespoons nutritional yeast
- 1 tablespoon soy sauce or tamari
- 1 tablespoon olive oil
- 4 whole-grain English muffins, halved and toasted
- Vegan mayo or your favorite plant-based spread
- Avocado slices
- Tomato slices
- Fresh spinach or arugula
- Salt and pepper to taste

Guidelines:
1. Marinate Tofu:
- Combine nutritional yeast, olive oil, and soy sauce or tamari in a shallow dish. Make sure the tofu slices are well coated by dipping them into the marinade. Give them at least ten to fifteen minutes to marinate.
2. Prepare Tofu:
- Turn up the heat to medium-high in a nonstick skillet. Simmer the marinated tofu slices until golden brown, 3 to 4 minutes per side.
3. Put the Sandwich Together:
Drizzle the toasted English muffins with vegan mayo or your favorite plant-based spread.
4. Layering the Ingredients:
 - Top each English muffin with a slice of tofu. - Add tomato, avocado, and fresh spinach or arugula slices on top.
5. Seasoning:
- Add pepper and salt to taste.
6. Top with the Other Half:
To finish off each English muffin sandwich, place the top half on top. This makes a full breakfast sandwich.
7. Serve Warm:
 - Present the vegan morning sandwiches in a warm state.

Cooking Time: - The sandwich assembly takes a few minutes, and the tofu needs about 6 to 8 minutes to cook. When marinating, the entire process should take about 15 minutes.

AVOCADO AND TOMATO TOAST

Ingredients:
- 2 slices of whole-grain bread
- 1 ripe avocado
- 1-2 medium tomatoes, thinly sliced
- Salt and pepper to taste
- Optional toppings: Red pepper flakes, balsamic glaze, or fresh herbs

Guidelines:
1. Toast the Bread:
- Toast the whole-grain bread slices until they are to your preference.
2. Prepare the avocado:
 Cut the ripe avocado in half, take out the pit, and scoop out the flesh into a bowl while the bread is toasting.
3. Mash Avocado:
Using a fork, mash the avocado until it has the consistency you want.
4. Spread Avocado on Toast:
- Evenly spread each slice of toasted bread with mashed avocado.
5. Add Tomato Slices on Top:
- Place the thinly sliced tomatoes over the avocado mash.
6. Season:
- Drizzle the tomato slices with salt and pepper, according to taste.
7. Optional Toppings:

- For extra flavor, you can optionally add toppings like fresh herbs, a drizzle of balsamic glaze, or red pepper flakes.
8. Serve Right Away:
- Serve the avocado and tomato toast as soon as possible to enjoy it fresh.

Cooking Time: - Preparing the avocado and tomatoes is quick, but toasting the bread takes a few minutes. The entire procedure ought to take five to ten minutes.

VEGAN BREAKFAST BURRITO

Ingredients:
- 1 cup firm tofu, crumbled
- 1 tablespoon olive oil
- 1/2 onion, diced
- 1 bell pepper, diced
- 1 small tomato, diced
- A cup of cooked and drained black beans
- 1 teaspoon ground cumin
- 1/2 teaspoon smoked paprika
- Salt and pepper to taste
- 4 large whole-grain or corn tortillas
- Vegan cheese (optional)
- Fresh salsa or avocado slices for topping

Guidelines:
1. Sauté Vegetables:
 - In a skillet over medium heat, heat the olive oil.
Add the bell pepper and chopped onion. Cook the
veggies until they become soft.
2. Add Tofu:
- Fill the skillet with crumbled tofu. Cook, stirring
occasionally, for 3–4 minutes.
3. Add the Beans and Spices:
 - Mix in the diced tomato, smoked paprika, ground
cumin, black beans, salt, and pepper. Cook for a
further two to three minutes, or until everything is
thoroughly mixed.
4. Warm Tortillas:
- Heat the tortillas in a different pan or right on the
stove.
5. Assemble Burritos: - Distribute evenly among the
tortillas the tofu and vegetable mixture.
6. Add Optional Ingredients:
- You can top the filling with vegan cheese if you'd
like.
7. Roll Burritos:
- To make a burrito, fold in the sides of each tortilla
and roll it tightly from the bottom.
Serve Warm:
 -Ensure that the vegan breakfast burritos are
served warm.
9. Add Avocado or Salsa on Top:
-To enhance the flavor, add slices of avocado or
fresh salsa.

Cooking Time: Depending on the speed and level of preparation, the vegan breakfast burrito can take anywhere from 15 to 20 minutes to cook through.

SWEET POTATO AND KALE HASH

Ingredients:
- 2 sweet potatoes, peeled and diced
- 1 bunch of kale, stems removed and chop the leaves
- 1 onion, diced
- 2 cloves garlic, minced
- 2 tablespoons olive oil
- 1 teaspoon smoked paprika
- 1/2 teaspoon ground cumin
- Salt and pepper to taste
- Optional toppings: Avocado slices, hot sauce, or a squeeze of lemon juice

Guidelines:
1. Prepare the ingredients:
chop the kale leaves, dice the onion, and peel and dice the sweet potatoes.
2. Sauté the onion and garlic:
- Heat the olive oil in a big skillet over medium heat. Add minced garlic and chopped onion. The onion should be sautéed until transparent.
3. Add Sweet Potatoes:
 - Fill the skillet with the chopped sweet potatoes. Stirring occasionally, cook for about 10 minutes or until they are slightly tender.
4. Add Spices:

-Drizzle the sweet potatoes with smoked paprika, ground cumin, salt, and pepper. To coat, thoroughly stir.

5. Add Kale:

- Fill the skillet with the chopped kale. Once the kale is tender and wilted, cook it for a further five to seven minutes, stirring to mix it with the sweet potatoes.

6. Modify Seasoning:

 - Taste the hash and make any required adjustments to the seasoning.

7. Serve Warm:

- Present the kale and sweet potato hash warmly.

8. Add Optional Toppings:

 -Squeeze some lemon juice, avocado slices, or hot sauce on top of the hash if you'd like.

Cooking Time: Depending on the size of the sweet potato dice and the desired level of tenderness, the sweet potato and kale hash will take about 20 to 25 minutes to cook in total.

CINNAMON APPLE OVERNIGHT OATS

Ingredients:
- 1/2 cup rolled oats
- 1/2 cup plant-based milk (almond, soy, or oat milk)
- 1/2 cup unsweetened applesauce
- 1/2 teaspoon ground cinnamon
- 1 tablespoon maple syrup or agave nectar
- 1/2 teaspoon vanilla extract
- 1 small apple, diced

- Optional toppings: Chopped nuts, raisins, or sliced apple

Instructions:
1. Combine Ingredients:
 - Place rolled oats, plant-based milk, applesauce, ground cinnamon, agave nectar or maple syrup, and vanilla extract in a jar or other lidded container.
2. Mix Well:
 Make sure all of the ingredients are well combined by giving them a good stir.
3. Add Diced Apple:
 - Fold the diced apple into the mixture of oats very gently.
4. Refrigerate Overnight:
 - Place a lid on the jar or container and place it in the refrigerator for a minimum of 4 hours, or better yet, overnight.
5. Stir Before Serving:
- Make sure the ingredients are thoroughly combined by giving the oats a good stir before serving.
6. Add Optional Toppings: You can add extra sliced apples, chopped nuts, or raisins as optional toppings.
7. Serve Cold: - Savor the overnight oats with cinnamon and apple cold out of the fridge.

 As the oats sit in the refrigerator, they take up the liquid and flavors. The overnight oats are ready to eat after 5 to 10 minutes of preparation.

SMOOTHIE BOWL

Ingredients:
- 1 frozen banana, sliced
- 1 cup frozen mixed berries (strawberries, blueberries, raspberries)
- 1/2 cup plant-based milk (almond, soy, or oat milk)
- 1 tablespoon nut butter
- Toppings: Granola, sliced fruit, chia seeds, shredded coconut

Guidelines:
1. Get Fruit Frozen:
   - Prepare the frozen mixed berries and slice and freeze the banana.
2. Blend Smoothie Base:
   - Place frozen banana slices, frozen mixed berries, plant-based milk, and nut butter into a blender.
3. Blend Until Smooth:
- Continue blending until a thick, smooth consistency is reached. To make sure everything is thoroughly mixed, you might need to pause and scrape down the sides.
4. Modify Consistency:
- If the smoothie is too thick, blend it again after adding a small amount more plant-based milk.
5. Pour into Bowl:
- Fill a bowl with the smoothie.
6. Add Toppings:
- Sprinkle granola, chopped fruit, chia seeds, shredded coconut, or any other preferred toppings on top of the smoothie bowl.

7. Serve Right Away: - Savor the smoothie bowl
right away while it's still cool and revitalizing.

Depending on your blender and the desired
smoothie thickness, the preparation and blending
take five to ten minutes.
To suit your tastes, feel free to get creative when it
comes to the toppings and ingredients. This tasty
and nourishing plant-based smoothie bowl is a
great choice for breakfast or a light snack.

PUMPKIN SPICE CHIA PUDDING

Ingredients:
- 1/4 cup chia seeds
- 1 cup plant-based milk (almond, soy, or coconut
milk)
- 1/2 cup canned pumpkin puree
- 2-3 tablespoons maple syrup or agave nectar
(adjust to taste)
- 1/2 teaspoon pumpkin pie spice (or a mix of
cinnamon, nutmeg, and cloves)
- 1/2 teaspoon vanilla extract
- Optional toppings: Chopped nuts, granola, or
whipped coconut cream

Guidelines:
1. Combine Ingredients:
- Mix plant-based milk, chia seeds, pumpkin puree,
agave nectar or maple syrup, pumpkin pie spice,
and vanilla extract in a bowl or jar.
2. Stir Well:

- Make sure the chia seeds are dispersed evenly and do not clump together by stirring the mixture thoroughly.

3. Chill:

- Place a lid on the bowl or jar and place it in the fridge for a minimum of three hours, or better yet, overnight. This enables the liquid to be absorbed by the chia seeds, giving the mixture a pudding-like consistency.

4. Stir Once More:

- Give the chia pudding another stir following the first refrigeration period. To get the right consistency, thin it out with a little more plant-based milk if it's too thick.

5. To serve, ladle the chia pudding with pumpkin spice into bowls or jars.

6. Add Toppings:

- If preferred, garnish with granola, chopped nuts, or a dollop of whipped coconut cream.

The main duration is while the chia seeds are refrigerated, waiting for them to absorb the liquid. For optimal results, allow for a minimum of 3 hours or overnight.

VEGAN WAFFLES

Ingredients:
- 1 1/2 cups all-purpose flour
- 2 tablespoons sugar
- 1 tablespoon baking powder
- 1/2 teaspoon salt

- 1 1/2 cups plant-based milk (almond, soy, or oat milk)
- 1/3 cup vegetable oil
- 1 teaspoon vanilla extract

Guidelines:
1. Preheat Waffle Iron:
- As directed by the manufacturer, preheat your waffle iron.
2. Combine Dry Ingredients:
- In a sizable mixing basin, blend together the sugar, baking powder, salt, and all-purpose flour.
3. Mix Wet Ingredients:
 - Place the plant-based milk, vegetable oil, and vanilla extract in a different bowl.
4. Combine Mixtures:
- Add the wet ingredients to the dry ingredients in a bowl. Mix until barely incorporated. Be careful to not overmix; some lumps are acceptable.
5. Prepare Waffles:
- If needed, lightly oil the waffle iron. Depending on the size of the waffle iron, pour the batter onto it and cover.
6. Cook in accordance with Waffle Iron Instructions:
- Prepare the waffles in accordance with your waffle iron's instructions. Usually, the cooking process takes four to six minutes.
7. Verify Doneness:
-Crisp and golden brown waffles are typically an indication that they are done. Your waffle iron may cause variations in the precise time.
8. Serve Warm:

-Remove the waffles from the iron with care, then serve them hot.

Cooking Time: Depending on your waffle iron, the usual cooking time for vegan waffles is 4 to 6 minutes. For optimal results, follow the manufacturer's instructions.

VEGAN FRENCH TOAST

Ingredients:
- 4 slices of your favorite plant-based bread
- 1 cup unsweetened plant-based milk (almond, soy, or oat milk)
- 2 tablespoons chickpea flour (besan)
- 1 tablespoon nutritional yeast
- 1 teaspoon ground flaxseed
- 1/2 teaspoon ground cinnamon
- 1/2 teaspoon vanilla extract
- Pinch of salt
- Coconut oil or vegan butter for cooking

Guidelines:
1. Get the batter ready:
-Mix plant-based milk, chickpea flour, nutritional yeast, ground flaxseed, ground cinnamon, vanilla extract, and a small amount of salt in a shallow bowl. Be sure to mix the batter very well.
2. Soak Bread:
- Coat both sides of each slice of bread with batter by dipping it in. Allow excess batter to drip off.
3. Heat Cooking Oil:

- Heat a skillet or non-stick pan over medium heat and add coconut oil or vegan butter.
4. Prepare the French toast by placing the soaked bread slices onto the heated skillet. Cook for 3–4 minutes on each side, or until crispy and golden brown.
5. Repeat:
 - Continue with the remaining bread slices, adjusting the pan's oil or vegan butter as necessary.
6. Present Warm:
 - Present the plant-based French toast warmly.
Cooking Time:
- Depending on the heat of your skillet and the desired level of crispiness, vegan French toast can be cooked for about 6 to 8 minutes.
5. Repeat:
 - Continue with the remaining bread slices, adjusting the pan's oil or vegan butter as necessary.
6. Present Warm:
 - Present the plant-based French toast warmly.

Cooking Time: -Depending on the heat of your skillet and the desired level of crispiness, vegan French toast can be cooked for about 6 to 8 minutes.

SAUTÉED SPINACH AND MUSHROOM BAGEL

Ingredients:
- 1 bagel, sliced and toasted
- 1 cup fresh spinach, washed and chopped
- 1 cup mushrooms, sliced
- 1 clove garlic, minced
- 1 tablespoon olive oil
- Salt and pepper to taste
- Optional toppings: Vegan cream cheese, avocado slices, or red pepper flakes

Instructions:
1. Sauté Mushrooms:
   - Heat olive oil in a pan over medium heat. Add sliced mushrooms and sauté for 3-5 minutes until they are tender and slightly browned.
2. Add Garlic and Spinach:
   - Add minced garlic to the mushrooms and sauté for an additional 1-2 minutes until fragrant. Then, add chopped spinach and sauté until wilted.
3. Season:
   - Season the sautéed mushrooms and spinach with salt and pepper to taste. Stir to combine.
4. Toast Bagel:
   - While sautéing the vegetables, toast the bagel slices until golden brown.
5. Assemble:
   - Spread vegan cream cheese on each toasted bagel half if desired.

6. Place the Sautéed Spinach and Mushroom Mixture on Top:
- Spoon the mixture onto the bagel halves.
7. Optional Toppings:
-For some taste explosion, top with avocado slices or a sprinkling of red pepper flakes.
8. Serve Warm:
- Present the warm bagel with sautéed spinach and mushrooms.

Cooking Time: Including preparation and bagel toasting, the sautéed spinach and mushrooms take about 10 to 15 minutes to cook in total.

CAULIFLOWER BREAKFAST BURRITOS

Ingredients:
- 2 cups cauliflower rice
- 1 tablespoon olive oil
- 1/2 onion, diced
- 1 bell pepper, diced
- 1 teaspoon ground cumin
- 1/2 teaspoon turmeric
- Salt and pepper to taste

Additional Burrito Ingredients:
- Whole-grain or corn tortillas
- Black beans, cooked and drained
- Avocado slices
- Salsa or pico de gallo
- Fresh cilantro, chopped (optional)

- Lime wedges for serving

Guidelines:
1. Sauté a "scramble" of cauliflower:
Heat the olive oil in a skillet over medium heat. Add the bell pepper and chopped onion. Sauté the veggies until they become tender.
2. Add the Cauliflower Rice:
 Fill the skillet with the cooked cauliflower rice. Cook, stirring occasionally, until the cauliflower is tender, about 5 to 7 minutes.
3. Season the cauliflower by sprinkling it with salt, pepper, turmeric, and ground cumin. Allow it to cook for a further two to three minutes after giving it a good stir.
4. Warm Tortillas:
 - Heat the tortillas in a different pan or right on the stove.
5. Put the burritos together by spooning the "scramble" of cauliflower onto each tortilla.
6. Add Black Beans and Avocado:
 - Place slices of avocado and black beans on top.
7. Add Cilantro and Salsa:
- Pour pico de gallo or salsa over the filling. If desired, add chopped cilantro.
8. Roll Burritos:
- To make a burrito, fold in the sides of each tortilla and roll it tightly.
9. Present with Lime Wedges:
Present the breakfast burritos made with cauliflower alongside lime wedges.

Cooking Time: - Including the time needed to sauté the vegetables and cook the cauliflower rice, the cauliflower "scramble" takes about 15 minutes to prepare.

CHAPTER THREE

LUNCH

VEGAN MINESTRONE SOUP

Ingredients:
- 1 tablespoon olive oil
- 1 onion, diced
- 2 carrots, peeled and sliced
- 2 celery stalks, sliced
- 3 cloves garlic, minced
- 1 can (15 oz) diced tomatoes
- 1 can (15 oz) washed kidney beans and drained
- 1 can (15 oz) washed cannellini beans and drained
- 6 cups vegetable broth
- 1 teaspoon dried oregano
- 1 teaspoon dried thyme
- 1 teaspoon dried rosemary
- 1 bay leaf
- 1 cup small pasta (e.g., elbow or ditalini)
- 2 cups chopped kale or spinach
- Salt and pepper to taste
- Vegan Parmesan cheese for topping (optional)

Guidelines:
1. Sauté Vegetables: - Place a large saucepan over medium heat with olive oil. Add the minced garlic, sliced celery, sliced carrots, and diced onion. Sauté the veggies till they get tender.

2. Add Beans and Tomatoes: - Add the kidney beans, cannellini beans, and diced tomatoes. Mix everything together.

3. Add Herbs and Broth: - Add the broth made of vegetables. Add the bay leaf, thyme, rosemary, and dried oregano. Mix thoroughly.

4. Bring to a Simmer: To enable the flavors to mingle, simmer the soup for fifteen to twenty minutes.

5. Prepare Pasta: - Include the tiny pasta in the broth and cook it until it reaches al dente, following the directions on the package.

6. Add Leafy Greens: - Cook the chopped spinach or kale for a further three to five minutes, or until the greens have wilted.

7. Season: Add salt and pepper to taste when preparing the minestrone soup. Take out the bay leaf.

8. To serve, spoon hot soup into individual bowls. Add some vegan Parmesan cheese on top if desired.

Cooking Time: Sautéing the vegetables and letting the soup simmer together take about 30 to 40 minutes of total cooking time for vegan minestrone soup.

VEGAN EGGPLANT PARMESAN

Ingredients:
For the Breaded Eggplant:
- 2 large eggplants, sliced into 1/2-inch rounds
- 1 cup all-purpose flour
- 1 cup breadcrumbs (ensure they're vegan)
- 1 cup plant-based milk (almond, soy, or oat)
- Salt and pepper to taste

For the Marinara Sauce:
- 2 cans crushed tomatoes (15 oz each)
- 2 cloves garlic, minced
- 1 teaspoon dried oregano
- 1 teaspoon dried basil
- 1/2 teaspoon onion powder
- Salt and pepper to taste

For Assembly:
- 2 cups vegan mozzarella cheese, shredded
- 1/2 cup vegan Parmesan cheese, grated
- Fresh basil or parsley for garnish (optional)
- Cooked spaghetti or your preferred pasta
(optional)

Guidelines:
1. Preheat Oven: - Set the oven's temperature to
375°F, or 190°C.
2. Prepare the eggplant: - To relieve extra moisture,
salt the eggplant slices and let them sit for about 15
minutes. Using paper towels, pat dry the areas.

3. Breading Station: - Assemble three shallow bowls: one containing flour, another containing plant-based milk, and a third containing breadcrumbs.

4. Bread the Eggplant: - Coat each slice of eggplant in breadcrumbs after dipping it in plant-based milk and flour. The breaded slices ought to be put on a baking pan.

5. Bake the Eggplant: - Bake the breaded eggplant slices for 20 to 25 minutes, or until they are crispy and golden brown, in a preheated oven.

6. To make the Marinara Sauce, put the crushed tomatoes, minced garlic, oregano, basil, onion powder, salt, and pepper in a pot.stirring occasionally for 15 to 20 minutes.

7. Put the Eggplant Parmesan together: Cover the bottom of a baking dish with marinara sauce. Place slices of roasted eggplant on top in a layer. Add some vegan Parmesan and mozzarella cheese on top. Iterate through the levels.

8. Last Layer: - Top with a heaping helping of vegan cheeses and a final layer of marinara sauce.

9. Bake: - Bake for 25 to 30 minutes, or until the cheese is bubbling and melted.

10. Garnish and Serve: - If preferred, garnish with fresh parsley or basil. Serve your favorite pasta, or cooked spaghetti, with the vegan eggplant parmesan.

Cooking Time:- The total cooking time for vegan Eggplant Parmesan is approximately 1 hour, including baking the eggplant, preparing the marinara sauce, and baking the assembled dish.

TOMATO BASIL QUINOA BOWL

Ingredients:
- 1 cup quinoa, rinsed
- 2 cups cherry tomatoes, halved
- 1 cup fresh basil leaves, chopped
- 1/4 cup balsamic glaze
- 1/4 cup extra-virgin olive oil
- Salt and pepper to taste
- Optional: Pine nuts or vegan feta for garnish

Guidelines:
1. Prepare the quinoa: Quinoa should be combined with two cups of water in a saucepan. After bringing to a boil, lower the heat, cover, and simmer the quinoa for 15 to 20 minutes, or until it is tender and the water has been absorbed. Using a fork, fluff.
2. Prepare the Cherry Tomatoes: Cut the cherry tomatoes in half while the quinoa is cooking.
3. Prepare the Basil Dressing: - In a small bowl, whisk together the extra-virgin olive oil, balsamic glaze, chopped fresh basil, salt, and pepper. To suit your taste, adjust.
4. Combine Ingredients: - Place the cooked quinoa and cherry tomatoes in a big bowl.
5. Add Basil Dressing: - Drizzle the quinoa and tomatoes with the basil dressing. For an even coat, toss.

6. Garnish: If preferred, top the tomato basil quinoa bowl with vegan feta or pine nuts.
7. Present: - Present the bowl of quinoa either warm or at room temperature.

Cooking Time: Including the time needed to cook the quinoa and make the dressing, the Tomato Basil Quinoa Bowl takes about 20 to 25 minutes to prepare.

VEGAN GREEK SALAD WRAP

Ingredients:
For the Greek Salad:
- 1 cup cherry tomatoes, halved
- 1 cucumber, diced
- 1/2 red onion, thinly sliced
- 1/2 cup Kalamata olives, pitted and sliced
- 1/2 cup vegan feta cheese, crumbled
- Fresh parsley, chopped
- Salt and pepper to taste

For the Lemon-Dill Dressing:
- 3 tablespoons extra-virgin olive oil
- 1 tablespoon red wine vinegar
- Juice of 1 lemon
- 1 teaspoon dried oregano
- 1 teaspoon dried dill
- Salt and pepper to taste

For Assembly:
- Whole-grain wraps or tortillas

- Hummus for spreading
- Fresh spinach leaves

Guidelines:
1. Assemble the Greek salad: Cherry tomatoes, cucumber, red onion, Kalamata olives, vegan feta cheese, and freshly cut parsley should all be combined in a bowl. Add pepper and salt for seasoning.
2. Prepare the Lemon-Dill Dressing: To make the dressing, combine the extra-virgin olive oil, red wine vinegar, lemon juice, dried dill, dried oregano, salt, and pepper in a small bowl.
3. Discard Salad Dressing:
   - Drizzle the Greek salad ingredients with the Lemon-Dill Dressing. Toss to evenly coat all parts.
4. Assemble Wraps: - Arrange tortillas or whole-grain wrappers. On each wrapper, spread a layer of hummus.
5. Add the Spinach: Top the hummus layer with a layer of fresh spinach leaves.
6. Top with Greek Salad combination: - Spoon the combination of Greek salad over the spinach layer onto the wrappers.
7. Fold and Roll: - To create a wrap, fold the sides of the wraps and then tightly roll them.
8. Slice and Serve: - You can choose to cut the wraps in half on the diagonal. Serve right away.

LENTIL SOUP

Ingredients:
- 1 cup dried green or brown lentils, washed and drained
- 1 onion, diced
- 2 carrots, diced
- 2 celery stalks, diced
- 3 cloves garlic, minced
- 1 can (15 oz) diced tomatoes
- 6 cups vegetable broth
- 1 teaspoon ground cumin
- 1 teaspoon ground coriander
- 1/2 teaspoon smoked paprika
- 1 bay leaf
- Salt and pepper to taste
- Fresh lemon juice (optional, for serving)
- Fresh parsley, chopped (for garnish)

Guidelines:
1. Sauté Vegetables: - In a big saucepan, cook chopped celery, carrots, and onion for five to seven minutes over medium heat, with a little water or olive oil added.
2. Add Spices and Garlic: - Add the minced garlic and sauté it for a further one to two minutes, or until it becomes aromatic. Add the smoked paprika, ground cumin, and ground coriander and stir.
3. Add Lentils and Tomatoes: - Fill the pot with chopped tomatoes (together with their juice), lentils

that have been rinsed, and vegetable broth. Mix thoroughly.

4. Boil and Simmer: - After bringing the soup to a boil, lower the heat, cover it, and simmer it for 25 to 30 minutes, or until the lentils are soft.

5. Season: Add salt and pepper to taste when preparing the lentil soup. A bay leaf might be added for taste.

6. Adjust Consistency (Optional): - You can add extra vegetable broth to the soup if it's too thick to your liking.

7. Take Out the Bay Leaf: - Before serving, dispose of the bay leaf.

8. To serve, spoon hot lentil soup into individual bowls. If preferred, drizzle a little freshly squeezed lemon juice over each serving.

9. Garnish: - Add freshly chopped parsley as a garnish.

Cooking Time: Including preparation and simmering, the entire cooking time for lentil soup is about 35 to 40 minutes.

VEGAN MEDITERRANEAN PIZZA

Ingredients:
For the Pizza Dough:
- Pre-made vegan pizza dough or store-bought crust
For the Toppings:
- 1/2 cup hummus (store-bought or homemade)
- 1 cup cherry tomatoes, halved

- 1/2 cup Kalamata olives, sliced
- 1/2 cup artichoke hearts, quartered
- 1/4 cup red onion, thinly sliced
- 1/4 cup sun-dried tomatoes, chopped
- 1/2 cup baby spinach leaves
- 1/2 cup vegan feta cheese, crumbled
- Olive oil for drizzling
- Fresh basil for garnish (optional)

Guidelines:
1. Preheat Oven: Follow the directions on the pizza dough package to preheat your oven.
2. Prepare the Pizza Dough: - Using a floured surface, roll out the pizza dough to the appropriate thickness.
3. Assemble the Pizza: - Place the rolled-out dough onto a baking sheet or pizza stone. As the pizza sauce, cover the dough with a layer of hummus.
4. Add Toppings: - Divide the vegan feta cheese, baby spinach, sun-dried tomatoes, red onion, artichoke hearts, and cherry tomatoes among the hummus's toppings.
5. Bake: - Bake the pizza in the oven that has been preheated, following the directions on the pizza dough, or until the toppings are cooked through and the crust has turned golden.
6. Drizzle with Olive Oil: - To add even more flavor, drizzle some olive oil over the pizza right out of the oven.
7. Garnish: - You can choose to add some fresh basil leaves on the pizza as a garnish.

8. Slice and Present: - Cut the Vegan
Mediterranean Pizza into slices and present it hot.

Cooking Duration: - Depending on which
pre-made pizza dough or crust you choose, the
Vegan Mediterranean Pizza's cooking time will vary.
It usually takes 15 to 20 minutes on medium to high
heat in the oven.

SPAGHETTI AGLIO E OLIO WITH BROCCOLI

Ingredients:
- 8 oz (about 225g) whole-grain spaghetti
- 1/4 cup olive oil
- 4 cloves garlic, thinly sliced
- 1/2 teaspoon red pepper flakes (adjust to taste)
- 1 head of broccoli, cut into florets
- Salt and black pepper to taste
- Fresh parsley, chopped, for garnish
- Vegan Parmesan cheese (optional)

Guidelines:
1. Prepare the pasta: - Cook the whole-grain
spaghetti until al dente, following the directions on
the package. Before draining, set aside about 1/2
cup of the pasta boiling water.
2. Blanch Broccoli: - Add the broccoli florets to the
boiling water during the final two to three minutes of
the spaghetti's cooking time. The broccoli will
blanch as a result. Rinse the broccoli and spaghetti
well.

3. Sauté Red pepper Flakes and Garlic: - Heat the olive oil in a big pan over medium heat. Add the red pepper flakes and the thinly sliced garlic. When the garlic is aromatic and just beginning to turn golden, sauté it for one to two minutes. Take care to prevent burning it.
4. Add Broccoli and pasta: - Add the broccoli and pasta, both drained, to the pan along with the red pepper flakes and garlic. Mix everything together to coat the broccoli and noodles in the delicious oil.
5. Season: - To taste, add salt and black pepper. To get the right consistency for your sauce, add a small amount of the pasta boiling water that was set aside if the pasta seems dry.
6. Garnish: - Sprinkle freshly cut parsley over the spaghetti aglio e olio. Add a dash of vegan Parmesan cheese if desired.
7. Serve: - Present the hot mixture of broccoli and noodles.

Cooking Time: Depending on how long the pasta cooks, the overall cooking time for spaghetti aglio e olio with broccoli is roughly 15-20 minutes.

CAPRESE SALAD WITH VEGAN MOZZARELLA

Ingredients:
- 2 large tomatoes, sliced
- 1 block (about 8 oz) vegan mozzarella, sliced
- Fresh basil leaves
- Balsamic glaze

- Extra-virgin olive oil
- Salt and pepper to taste

Guidelines:
1. Get the vegan mozzarella and tomatoes ready.
   - Cut the vegan mozzarella and tomatoes into uniform, medium-thick slices.
2. Assemble Salad: - On a serving platter or individual plates, alternately arranged tomato and vegan mozzarella slices.
3. Add the Basil Leaves: - Place a few fresh basil leaves in between the slices of mozzarella and tomato.
4. Drizzle with Olive Oil and Balsamic Glaze: - Drizzle the tomato and mozzarella slices with extra-virgin olive oil and balsamic glaze.
5. Season: - Drizzle the entire salad with salt and pepper, to taste.
6. Serve: - Present the Caprese Salad right away, topped with vegan mozzarella.

Savor this cool, plant-based caprese salad.The vivid aromas of tomatoes and fresh basil are complemented by the creamy texture of vegan mozzarella in this vegan take on the traditional Caprese salad, which perfectly captures the essence of the original. It is delicious and filling as an appetizer or meal.

VEGAN SUSHI ROLLS

Ingredients:
For Sushi Rice:
- 2 cups sushi rice
- 1/3 cup rice vinegar
- 2 tablespoons sugar
- 1 teaspoon salt

For Vegan Sushi Rolls:
- Nori (seaweed) sheets
- Sushi rice (prepared using the ingredients above)
- Avocado, sliced
- Cucumber, julienned
- Carrot, julienned
- Red bell pepper, julienned
- Extra-firm tofu, sliced into thin strips
- Soy sauce or tamari for dipping
- Pickled ginger and wasabi for serving

Guidelines:
1. Prepare the Sushi Rice: - Run cold water over the sushi rice until it flows clear. Follow the directions on the package to cook the rice. Rice vinegar, sugar, and salt should be heated in a small saucepan over low heat until the sugar is dissolved. Once done, mix in the seasoned rice vinegar and set aside to cool.
2. Prepare the ingredients: - Cut the tofu and veggies into thin, even strips.

3. Assembly: - On a spotlessly surface, place a bamboo sushi rolling mat. Arrange a nori sheet on the mat, shiny side down.

4. Spread Rice: - Using wet hands, cover the nori with a thin coating of sushi rice, leaving the top half an inch or so uncovered.

5. Add Fillings: - Line the bottom border of the rice with a few slices of avocado, cucumber, carrot, tofu, or any other filling you choose.

6. Roll: - Roll the nori and rice over the fillings, gently pressing with the bamboo mat. Apply a little water to seal the edge.

7. Slice: - Cut the sushi roll into bite-sized pieces using a sharp, moist knife.

8. Repeat: - Carry out the same procedure with the remaining fillings and nori sheets.

9. Present: - Present the vegan sushi rolls accompanied by wasabi, pickled ginger, and soy sauce.

PESTO ZOODLES

Ingredients:
- 4 medium zucchini, spiralized into noodles
- 1 cup fresh basil leaves
- 1/2 cup nuts (pine nuts, almonds, or walnuts)
- 2 cloves garlic
- 1/2 cup nutritional yeast (for a cheesy flavor, optional)
- 1/2 cup extra-virgin olive oil
- Salt and pepper to taste
- Cherry tomatoes, halved (optional, for garnish)

- Vegan Parmesan cheese (optional, for garnish)

Guidelines:
1. To make Zoodles, spiralize the zucchini using a spiralizer into noodles. If you don't have a spiralizer, you may still make thin strips by using a vegetable or julienne peeler.
2. To make the pesto sauce, pulse the fresh basil, almonds, garlic, and nutritional yeast (if using) in a food processor. Pulse until chopped finely.
3. Add Olive Oil: To make a smooth pesto sauce, gradually add the extra-virgin olive oil while the food processor is operating. To taste, add salt and pepper for seasoning.
4. Toss Zoodles with Pesto: - Place the zucchini noodles in a big bowl and toss them until thoroughly coated with the freshly created pesto sauce.
5. Garnish: If preferred, garnish with vegan Parmesan cheese and cherry tomatoes that have been cut in half.
6. Serve: - Present the Pesto Zoodles right now.

Cooking Time: 5 to 10 minutes (depending on your equipment and level of competence) for spiralizing zucchini.
- 5 minutes to make the pesto sauce.
- Five minutes for tossing and garnishing.
Cooking time total: about 15 to 20 minutes

STIR-FRIED TOFU AND VEGGIES

Ingredients:
- 1 tablespoon cornstarch
2 tablespoons sesame oil
1 tablespoon vegetable oil
- 3 chopped cloves of garlic
- 14 lb (400g) firm tofu, pressed and diced;
-1 bell pepper, thinly sliced; one carrot, julienned
1 tablespoon grated ginger; one cup broccoli florets
- 1 cup blanched snap peas
- 2 sliced green onions
- Optional sesame seeds for garnish
- Prepared cooked quinoa or brown rice for serving

Guidelines:
1. Tofu preparation: Press the tofu to squeeze out extra water, then chop it into cubes. Toss the tofu cubes with cornstarch and soy sauce in a bowl until well covered.
2. Stir-Fry Tofu: - Heat sesame oil in a large skillet or wok over medium-high heat. When the tofu cubes are brown and crispy on both sides, add them and pan-fry. Take out the tofu and place it aside.
3. Stir-Fry Vegetables: - Pour vegetable oil into the same pan. Fry the ginger and garlic until aromatic. Add the snap peas, broccoli, carrot, and bell pepper. Stir-fry the vegetables for 4–5 minutes and until they are crisp-tender.

4. Mix Tofu and Vegetables: - Return the pan-fried tofu to the pan along with the vegetables. Mix everything until thoroughly incorporated.
5. Add the green onions last: - Add the chopped onions and toss for a minute more.
6. Garnish and Serve: - If preferred, garnish with sesame seeds. Serve the cooked quinoa or brown rice with the stir-fried tofu and veggies.

Cooking time: 15 to 20 minutes for pressing tofu (optional, but recommended for improved texture).
- Five minutes for tofu preparation and marinating.
- Tofu pan-fried for 10 to 15 minutes.
- Stir-fry veggies for 5 to 7 minutes.
Cooking time total: about 35–47 minutes

CAULIFLOWER BUFFALO WINGS SALAD

Ingredients
 Buffalo Wings with Cauliflower:
- 1 medium-sized head of cauliflower, divided into pieces
- 3/4 cup all-purpose flour (for a gluten-free alternative, use chickpea flour)
- 3/4 cup of plant-based milk, without sugar
- 1 teaspoon powdered garlic
– 1 teaspoon powdered onion
- 1/2 tsp smoked paprika
- 1 cup breadcrumbs (or panko breadcrumbs for added crispiness)
 - Salt and pepper to taste

- 1 cup of homemade or store-bought buffalo sauce
For Salad:
- Mixed salad greens (lettuce, spinach, arugula, etc.)
- Cherry tomatoes, halved
- Cucumber, sliced
- Avocado, sliced
- Vegan ranch dressing for drizzling

Guidelines:
1. Preheat Oven: Set the oven's temperature to 450°F, or 230°C.
2. Assemble the cauliflower wings: Combine the flour, plant-based milk, smoked paprika, onion and garlic powders, salt, and pepper in a bowl. To get a uniform coating, dip each cauliflower floret into the batter and then roll it in breadcrumbs. The coated florets should be put on a baking sheet.
3. Bake the cauliflower wings: - Bake the cauliflower for 20 to 25 minutes, or until it's crispy and golden.
4. Drizzle with Buffalo Sauce: - In a saucepan, warm up the buffalo sauce over low heat while the cauliflower bakes. After cooking, toss the roasted cauliflower florets in the buffalo sauce until well coated.
5. Assemble the Salad: - Combine the avocado slices, cherry tomatoes, cucumber, and mixed salad greens in a big bowl.
6. Add Cauliflower Wings on Top: - Arrange the salad on top of the buffalo cauliflower wings.

7. Drizzle with Vegan Ranch: - Pour vegan ranch dressing over the salad.
8. Serve: - Present the Buffalo Wings Salad with cauliflower right away.

Cooking Time: Approximately 30 to 40 minutes are needed to cook the cauliflower buffalo wings and assemble the salad.

VEGAN BBQ JACKFRUIT SANDWICH

Ingredients:
 1 cup barbecued jackfruit
- 2 20-oz cans of young green jackfruit in brine, each after draining and rinsing
- 1 cup of homemade or store-bought barbecue sauce
- 1 tablespoon each of olive oil and garlic powder
- 1 tsp of paprika with smoke
To taste, add salt and pepper.

Regarding Sandwich:
- Whole-grain rolls or buns
- Coleslaw (prepared or purchased from the shop)
- Pickles (optional)
- Optional vegan mayonnaise

Guidelines:
1. Get the jackfruit ready:
   - To give the jackfruit the texture of pulled flesh, shred it with a fork or your hands.

2. Sauté the Jackfruit: - Heat the olive oil in a pan over medium heat. Add the smoked paprika, garlic powder, salt, and pepper along with the shredded jackfruit. When the jackfruit starts to brown, sauté it for three to five minutes.

3. Add BBQ Sauce: - Drizzle the jackfruit with the barbecue sauce and mix to coat. Simmer on low heat for a further ten to fifteen minutes so the jackfruit can absorb the spices.

4. Assemble the Sandwich: Toast the bread rolls or whole-grain buns. Spoon a large amount of the Barbecued jackfruit onto the lower half.

5. Top with Coleslaw and Pickles: To add extra crunch and freshness, top with coleslaw and pickles.

6. Optional: Vegan Mayonnaise: - If preferred, spread vegan mayonnaise over the upper portion of the bun.

7. Serve: - Quickly serve the vegan BBQ jackfruit sandwich by covering it with the top half of the bun.

Cooking Time: - It will take about 20 to 25 minutes to cook the vegan BBQ jackfruit and put the sandwich together.

THAI COCONUT CURRY SOUP

Ingredients:
- 1 tablespoon coconut oil
- 1 sliced onion
- 2 julienned carrots
- 1 sliced red bell pepper

- 1 can (14 oz) coconut milk
 - 2 tablespoons red curry paste
- 1 tablespoon soy sauce
- 3 cups vegetable broth
- One tablespoon of lime juice
- To garnish, fresh cilantro

Guidelines:
1. Saute the bell pepper, onions, and carrots in a pot with coconut oil.
2. Include the lime juice, soy sauce, coconut milk, red curry paste, and vegetable broth.
3. Simmer for ten to fifteen minutes.
4. Before serving, garnish with fresh cilantro.

CREAMY BROCCOLI AND POTATO SOUP

Ingredients:
- 2 cups chopped broccoli florets
 - 2 diced and peeled potatoes
 - 1 chopped onion
 – 3 cups vegetable stock
 – 1 cup almond milk without sugar
- Two tablespoons of dietary yeast
- Season with salt and pepper - Garnish with chives

Guidelines:
1. Put the potatoes, broccoli, onion, and vegetable broth in a pot.
2. Simmer the veggies for tenderness.

3. Return the soup to the pot after blending it until it's smooth.

4. Add nutritional yeast, salt, pepper, and almond milk.

5. Before serving, fully heat and add chives as a garnish.

Cooking Time:

- 5 to 7 minutes for sautéing veggies.

Vegetables should be simmered for 15 to 20 minutes until soft.

5 minutes for blending and adding back to the pot.

- Last heating for five to seven minutes, using almond milk and nutritional yeast.

The entire cooking process takes about 30 to 40 minutes.

PUMPKIN AND LENTIL CURRY

Ingredients:

- 1 cup washed and dried red lentils
- 2 cups diced butternut squash or pumpkin
- 1 finely chopped onion
- 2 minced garlic cloves
- One tablespoon of grated ginger
- 1 14-ounce can of coconut milk
- 1 14-oz can of chopped tomatoes
- 2 tsp curry powder
- 1/2 teaspoon chili powder (adjust to taste)
- 1 teaspoon each of turmeric, cumin, and coriander

Season with salt and pepper

- Garnish with fresh cilantro
 - Serve with cooked brown rice or quinoa

Guidelines:
1. Sauté Aromatics: - In a large saucepan, sauté minced garlic, grated ginger, and chopped onions until the ginger is tender.
2. Add Spices: - Add chili powder, curry powder, turmeric, cumin, and coriander. Coat the aromatics with the spices by stirring them.
3. Add Pumpkin and Lentils: - Fill the pot with diced pumpkin (or butternut squash), diced tomatoes, and coconut milk once the lentils have been washed. Blend thoroughly.
4. Simmer: - After bringing the mixture to a boil, lower the heat, and simmer it for 20 to 25 minutes, or until the pumpkin and lentils are soft.
5. Season: - Add salt and pepper to taste when preparing the curry. Taste and adjust the seasonings.
6. Garnish and Serve: - Add fresh cilantro to the Pumpkin and Lentil Curry. Serve with cooked quinoa or brown rice.

Cooking Time: Depending on how soft the lentils and pumpkin are, the overall cooking time for Pumpkin and Lentil Curry is about 30 to 40 minutes.

SWEET POTATO AND BLACK BEAN QUESADILLA

Ingredients:
- 1 large sweet potato, peeled and diced
- 1 can (15 oz) black beans, washed and rinsed
- 1 teaspoon olive oil
- 1 onion, finely chopped
- 2 cloves garlic, minced
- 1 teaspoon ground cumin
- 1 teaspoon chili powder
- Salt and pepper to taste
- 4 big whole wheat or corn tortillas
- 1 cup vegan cheese, shredded (cheddar or Mexican blend)
- Fresh cilantro, chopped (optional)
- Salsa or guacamole for serving

Guidelines:
1. Sweet potato roast: Set oven temperature to 400°F, or 200°C. Add salt, pepper, and olive oil to the chopped sweet potato. Roast in the oven until soft, about 20 minutes.
2. Sauté Onion and Garlic: - Finely cut the onion and mince the garlic, then sauté them in a skillet until they become soft.
3. Add Black Beans and Spices: - Fill the pan with black beans, chili powder, ground cumin, salt, and pepper. Simmer for five more minutes.
4. Assemble the quesadillas by layering the roasted sweet potato, vegan cheese, chopped cilantro, if

using, and the black bean mixture on one side of each tortilla. Half the tortillas should be folded.
5. Cook Quesadillas: - Cook each quesadilla for two to three minutes on each side, or until the cheese has melted and the tortilla is golden. This can be done in a skillet over medium heat.
6. Present: - Cut the quesadillas into wedges and present them alongside guacamole or salsa.

Cooking Time: - Roasting the sweet potatoes and assembling/cooking the quesadillas add about 30 to 35 minutes to the overall cooking time for Sweet Potato and Black Bean Quesadillas.

MEXICAN QUINOA SALAD

Ingredients:
- 1 cup quinoa, rinsed
- 2 cups water or vegetable broth
- 1 can (15 oz) black beans, washed and rinsed
- 1 cup kernels corn (fresh or frozen)
- 1 bell pepper, diced
- 1 cup cherry tomatoes, halved
- 1/2 red onion, finely chopped
- 1/4 cup fresh cilantro, chopped
- 1 avocado, diced
- Juice of 2 limes
- 2 tablespoons olive oil
- 1 teaspoon ground cumin
- 1 teaspoon chili powder
- Salt and pepper to taste
- Optional: Jalapeño slices for extra spice

Guidelines:
1. Prepare Quinoa: - Put quinoa and water or vegetable broth in a pot. After bringing to a boil, lower the heat to low, cover, and simmer the quinoa for 15 to 20 minutes, or until it is tender and the liquid has been absorbed. Using a fork, fluff.
2. Prepare the Vegetables: - Combine the bell pepper, cherry tomatoes, red onion, cilantro, black beans, and corn in a big bowl.
3. Prepare the Dressing: - Combine the lime juice, olive oil, chili powder, ground cumin, salt, and pepper in a small bowl.
4. Mix and Toss: - Include the cooked quinoa in the vegetable bowl. After adding the dressing to the salad, toss everything until thoroughly mixed.
5. Add Avocado: - Fold in the cubed avocado gently.
6. Chill (Optional): To enable the flavors to blend, place the salad in the refrigerator for a minimum of half an hour.

Cooking Time: - Cooking the quinoa and preparing the vegetables take about 20 to 25 minutes altogether when making Mexican Quinoa Salad.

VEGAN BLT SANDWICH

Ingredients:
- 8 slices whole-grain bread
- 1 cup cherry tomatoes, sliced
- 1 head of lettuce, washed and torn into pieces

- 1 package (about 8 oz) tempeh bacon or smoked tofu, thinly sliced
- 1 avocado, sliced
- Vegan mayonnaise
- Dijon mustard
- Salt and pepper to taste
- Optional: Pickles for added flavor

Guidelines:
1. Cook the Tempeh Bacon or Smoked Tofu
: - Cook the pieces of tempeh bacon or smoked tofu in a pan over medium heat until they are crispy on both sides. Usually, this takes five to seven minutes.
2. Prepare the Bread: - Toast the slices of whole-grain bread until they are as crispy as you like.
3. Assemble Sandwiches: - Spread each slice of bread with vegan mayonnaise on one side. Brush the slices with Dijon mustard on half of them.
4. Arrange Ingredients: - Arrange cherry tomatoes, lettuce, avocado slices, tempeh bacon or smoked tofu, and salt and pepper to taste on the slices dipped in mayonnaise. Drizzle the remaining slices of bread with Dijon mustard.
5. Optional: Top with Pickles: - Garnish your sandwich with pickles for an added crunch.
6. Serve: - Cut the sandwiches in half lengthwise and present them right away.

Cooking Time: - Cooking the tempeh bacon or smoked tofu and toasting the bread will take about ten to fifteen minutes overall when making the vegan BLT sandwich.

CHICKPEA AND SPINACH CURRY

Ingredients:
- 1 can (15 oz) chickpeas, washed and raised
- 1 onion, finely chopped
- 2 cloves garlic, minced
- 1-inch piece of ginger, grated
- 1 can (14 oz) diced tomatoes
- 1 can (14 oz) coconut milk
- 1 tablespoon curry powder
- 1 teaspoon ground cumin
- 1 teaspoon ground coriander
- 1/2 teaspoon turmeric
- 1/2 tsp cayenne pepper (adjust to taste)
- Salt and pepper to taste
- 4 cups fresh spinach, raised and chopped
- 1 tablespoon vegetable oil
- Fresh cilantro for garnish
- Cooked rice or naan for serving

Guidelines:
1. Sauté Aromatics: - Heat vegetable oil in a large pan over medium heat. Chop the onions and sauté them until tender.
2. Add Garlic and Ginger: - Fill the pan with grated ginger and minced garlic. Sauté until aromatic, one or two more minutes.
3. Add the Spices: - Mix in the curry powder, cayenne pepper, turmeric, ground coriander, cumin,

and pepper. Toasted the spices for one to two minutes.

4. Mix Tomatoes and Chickpeas: - Transfer chopped tomatoes and chickpeas, along with their juices, to a pan. Mix thoroughly to blend.

5. Simmer: After adding the coconut milk, simmer the curry for 15 to 20 minutes to allow the spices to seep into the chickpeas and the flavors to combine.

6. Add the spinach: Cook the chopped spinach until it wilts by stirring it in.

7. Modify Seasoning: - If necessary, taste and adjust the seasoning.

8. To serve, arrange the cooked rice or naan alongside the Chickpea and Spinach Curry. Add fresh cilantro as a garnish.

Cooking Time: Approximately 25 to 30 minutes are needed to prepare the chickpea and spinach curry.

CHAPTER FOUR

DINNER

VEGAN SPAGHETTI BOLOGNESE

Ingredients:
- 1 lb (about 450g) whole-grain or lentil spaghetti
- 1 tablespoon olive oil
- 1 large onion, finely chopped
- 2 carrots, grated
- 2 celery stalks, finely chopped
- 3 cloves garlic, minced
- 1 can (14 oz) lentils, drained and rinsed (or cooked green or brown lentils)
- 1 can (14 oz) crushed tomatoes
- 2 tablespoons tomato paste
- 1 teaspoon dried oregano
- 1 teaspoon dried basil
- 1/2 teaspoon dried thyme
- Salt and pepper to taste
- Red pepper flakes (optional, for heat)
- Fresh basil or parsley for garnish
- Vegan Parmesan or nutritional yeast for topping

Guidelines:

1. Prepare the spaghetti: - Cook the spaghetti until al dente, following the directions on the package. After draining, set away.

2. Sauté Vegetables: - Heat olive oil in a large pan over medium heat. Add the chopped celery, chopped onions, and shredded carrots. Sauté the vegetables for 5 to 7 minutes, or until they are tender.

3. Add Garlic and Lentils: - Fill the pan with the minced garlic and the drained lentils. Simmer for two more minutes.

4. Tomato Base: - Add salt, pepper, crushed tomatoes, tomato paste, dried thyme, dry basil, and dried oregano, if using. Simmer the mixture for a while.

5. Simmer: - Turn down the heat to low, cover, and simmer, stirring now and again, for at least twenty to twenty-five minutes. As a result, the flavors can combine.

6. Modify Seasoning: - Taste and make any necessary adjustments to the seasoning. You can thin it out with a small amount of water or veggie broth.

7. Present: - Arrange the cooked spaghetti on top of the vegan Bolognese. Top with nutritional yeast or vegan Parmesan cheese and garnish with fresh basil or parsley.

 Cooking Time: Including preparation and simmering, the entire cooking time for Plant-Based Vegan Spaghetti Bolognese is about 30 to 40 minutes.

LEMON HERB QUINOA SALAD

Ingredients:
- 1 cup quinoa, rinsed
- 2 cups water or vegetable broth
- 1 cucumber, diced
- 1 cup cherry tomatoes, halved
- 1 bell pepper (any color), diced
- 1/4 cup red onion, finely chopped
- 1/4 cup fresh parsley, chopped
- 1/4 cup fresh mint, chopped
- 1/3 cup extra-virgin olive oil
- Juice of 2 lemons
- Salt and pepper to taste
- Optional: Kalamata olives or vegan feta for extra flavor

Guidelines:
1. Prepare the quinoa: Quinoa should be combined with water or vegetable broth in a saucepan. After bringing to a boil, lower the heat to low, cover, and simmer the quinoa for 15 to 20 minutes, or until it is tender and the liquid has been absorbed. Using a fork, fluff and allow to cool.
2. Prepare the Herbs and Vegetables: Finely chop the red onion, dice the bell pepper, dice the cucumber, cut the cherry tomatoes in half, and chop the fresh parsley and mint.

3. Prepare Dressing: - To make the dressing, whisk together olive oil, lemon juice, salt, and pepper in a small bowl.
4. Combine Ingredients: - Place cooked and cooled quinoa, sliced cucumber, cherry tomatoes cut in half, diced bell pepper, chopped red onion, parsley, and mint in a big bowl.
5. Dress the Salad: - Drizzle the salad with the lemon and herb dressing, then toss to fully incorporate.
6. Optional Additions: - For added taste, feel free to incorporate vegan feta or Kalamata olives.
7. Chill (Optional): To let the flavors blend, place the salad in the fridge for at least half an hour before serving.

Cooking Time: Including the time needed to cook the quinoa and prep the veggies, the Lemon Herb Quinoa Salad takes about 20 to 25 minutes to cook in total.

VEGAN BUDDHA BOWL

Ingredients:
For the Bowl:
- 1 cup cooked quinoa or rice
- 1 cup roasted sweet potatoes, cubed
- 1 cup steamed broccoli florets
- 1/2 cup shredded carrots
- 1/2 cup red cabbage, thinly sliced
- 1/2 cup cucumber, sliced
- 1/2 avocado, sliced

- 1/4 cup edamame, cooked
- for garnish Sesame seeds and green onions

For the Tahini Dressing:
- 3 tablespoons tahini
- 2 tablespoons soy sauce or tamari
- 1 tablespoon maple syrup
- 1 tablespoon rice vinegar
- 1 teaspoon sesame oil
- 1 clove garlic, minced
- Water to thin as needed

Guidelines:
1. Cook Rice or Quinoa: - Follow the directions on the package to prepare one cup of rice or quinoa.
2. Bake Sweet Potatoes: - Set oven temperature to 400°F, or 200°C. Combine salt, pepper, and olive oil with the cubed sweet potatoes. Roast for 20 to 25 minutes, or until soft and brown.
3. Steam Broccoli: Steam broccoli florets for five to seven minutes, or until they are soft but still have a brilliant green color.
4. Prepare the Other Vegetables: - Slice the cucumber, shave the red cabbage, shred the carrots, and prepare the avocado and edamame.
5. Assemble the Buddha Bowl by placing the quinoa, edamame, cucumber, avocado, steamed broccoli, shredded carrots, red cabbage, and roasted sweet potatoes in a bowl.
6. Prepare the Tahini Dressing: - Combine the tahini, soy sauce, maple syrup, rice vinegar, sesame oil, and minced garlic in a small bowl.

Water can be added as needed to get the right consistency.

7. Drizzle Dressing: Cover the Buddha Bowl with a drizzle of tahini dressing.

8. Garnish: Add green onions and sesame seeds as garnish.

Cooking Time: Depending on how the quinoa or rice is cooked and how the sweet potatoes are roasted, the entire cooking time for a vegan Buddha bowl is between 25 to 30 minutes.

VEGAN SPINACH AND ARTICHOKE

Ingredients:
- 1 can (14 oz) artichoke hearts, drained and chopped
- 2 cups fresh spinach, chopped
- 1/2 cup vegan mayonnaise
- 1/2 cup vegan cream cheese
- 1/2 cup nutritional yeast
- 1/4 cup unsweetened almond milk (or any plant-based milk)
- 3 cloves garlic, minced
- 1 teaspoon onion powder
- 1/2 teaspoon garlic powder
- 1/2 teaspoon dried basil
- 1/2 teaspoon dried thyme
- Salt and pepper to taste
- Vegan shredded cheese for topping (optional)
- Fresh parsley for garnish

- Sliced baguette, tortilla chips, or vegetable sticks for serving

Guidelines:
1. Preheat Oven: - Set the oven's temperature to 375°F, or 190°C.
2. Combine Ingredients: - Add chopped artichoke hearts, chopped spinach, vegan mayonnaise, vegan cream cheese, nutritional yeast, almond milk, minced garlic, onion powder, garlic powder, dried basil, dried thyme, salt, and pepper to a large mixing bowl. Until all components are mixed, thoroughly mix.
3. Transfer to Baking Dish: - Evenly spread out the mixture on a baking dish.
4. Bake: - Bake for about 25 to 30 minutes in a preheated oven, or until the dip is well heated and the sides turn brown.
5. Optional Topping: - For a melted, cheesy finish, sprinkle vegan shredded cheese on top during the final five minutes of baking.
6. Garnish and Serve: Take out of the oven, sprinkle with fresh parsley, and serve warm with tortilla chips, vegetable sticks, or sliced baguette.

Cooking Time: - Plant-Based Vegan Spinach and Artichoke Dip takes about 25 to 30 minutes to cook in total.

VEGAN TERIYAKI TEMPEH BOWL

Ingredients:
For Teriyaki Tempeh:

- 1 package (about 8 oz) tempeh, sliced
- 1/4 cup soy sauce or tamari
- 2 tablespoons maple syrup or agave nectar
- 1 tablespoon rice vinegar
- 1 teaspoon sesame oil
- 1 teaspoon grated ginger
- 2 cloves garlic, minced

For the Bowl:
- 2 cups cooked brown rice or quinoa
- 1 cup broccoli florets, steamed
- 1 medium carrot, julienned
- 1/2 red bell pepper, thinly sliced
- 1/2 cup edamame, cooked
- Sesame seeds and green onions for garnish
- Optional: Sliced avocado for topping

Guidelines:
1. Make the Teriyaki Sauce: To make the teriyaki sauce, combine the soy sauce or tamari, rice vinegar, sesame oil, grated ginger, and chopped garlic in a bowl.
2. Marinate the Tempeh: - Spread half of the teriyaki sauce over the sliced Tempeh that you have placed in a shallow dish. Give it a minimum of 15 to 30 minutes to marinate.

3. Cook the Tempeh: - Cook the marinated tempeh slices in a pan over medium heat for 3–4 minutes on each side, or until golden brown. While cooking, brush with more teriyaki sauce.

4. Prepare the Vegetables: Steam the broccoli florets and boil the edamame as directed on the package. Slice the red bell pepper thinly and julienne the carrots.

5. Assemble Bowl: - Arrange cooked brown rice or quinoa, sliced red bell pepper, steamed broccoli, julienned carrots, and edamame in serving bowls.

6. Add Teriyaki Tempeh: - Top the bowl with the cooked slices of teriyaki tempeh.

7. Add a garnish by tossing chopped green onions and sesame seeds on top. If desired, add sliced avocado.

8. To serve, quickly pour the leftover teriyaki sauce over the bowl.

Cooking Time: Including the tempeh's marinating period, the Plant-Based Vegan Teriyaki Tempeh Bowl takes about 30 to 40 minutes to cook in total.

VEGAN GNOCCHI WITH TOMATO BASIL SAUCE

Ingredients:
- 1 package (about 16 oz) vegan gnocchi
- 2 tablespoons olive oil
- 3 cloves garlic, minced
- 1 can (28 oz) crushed tomatoes
- 1 teaspoon dried oregano

- 1 teaspoon dried basil
- 1/2 teaspoon red pepper flakes (optional, for heat)
- Salt and pepper to taste
- Fresh basil leaves for garnish
- Vegan Parmesan or nutritional yeast for topping

Guidelines:
1. Prepare the Gnocchi: - Follow the directions on the package to prepare the vegan gnocchi. They cook quickly, usually just a few minutes, and are done when they float to the top.
2. Make Tomato Basil Sauce: - Heat olive oil in a skillet over medium heat. Once aromatic, add the minced garlic and sauté it for one to two minutes.
3. Add Crushed Tomatoes and Seasonings: - Add salt, pepper, dried oregano, dried basil, and red pepper flakes, if using, to the crushed tomatoes. Mix thoroughly to blend.
4. Simmer Sauce: - Lower the heat to a simmer and leave the sauce for fifteen to twenty minutes, so that the flavors may combine and the sauce can thicken.
5. Mix Gnocchi and Sauce:-Drain the cooked gnocchi and mix it with the tomato-basil sauce. Toss the gnocchi gently to coat them with sauce.
6. Garnish and Serve:-Place the vegan gnocchi in bowls and top with nutritional yeast or vegan Parmesan cheese. Garnish with fresh basil leaves.

Cooking Time: - Cooking the gnocchi and simmering the sauce together takes about 20 to 25 minutes for Plant-Based Vegan Gnocchi with Tomato Basil Sauce.

VEGAN STUFFED MUSHROOM

Ingredients:
- 16-20 large cremini or button mushrooms, cleaned and stems removed
- 1 cup breadcrumbs (ensure they are vegan)
- 1/2 cup finely chopped onion
- 1/2 cup finely chopped red bell pepper
- 2 cloves garlic, minced
- 1/4 cup chopped fresh parsley
- 1/4 cup nutritional yeast
- 2 tablespoons olive oil
- 1 tablespoon soy sauce or tamari
- 1 teaspoon dried thyme
- Salt and pepper to taste
- Vegan Parmesan for topping (optional)

Guidelines:
1. Preheat Oven: - Set the oven's temperature to 375°F, or 190°C.
2. Prepare the Mushrooms: - Chop the mushrooms finely after removing the stems. The mushroom caps should be set aside.
3. Sauté the Vegetables: - Heat the olive oil in a pan over medium heat. Add the minced garlic, bell pepper, and onion, chopped. Sauté the veggies till they get tender.
4. Get the stuffing mixture ready. Add the chopped mushroom stems, breadcrumbs, chopped parsley,

nutritional yeast, soy sauce or tamari, dried thyme, salt, and pepper to a bowl with the sautéed vegetables. To create a cohesive stuffing mixture, thoroughly mix.

5. Stuff Mushrooms: - Load the stuffing mixture into each mushroom cap, pressing it down a little bit.

6. Bake: - Put the stuffed mushrooms on a baking sheet and bake for 20 to 25 minutes, or until the stuffing is brown and the mushrooms are soft.

7. Optional Garnish: - For a cheesy final touch, feel free to sprinkle vegan Parmesan over the top in the final few minutes of baking.

8. Serve: After they are cooked, take them out of the oven and allow them to cool a little before slicing.

Cooking Time: Including preparation and baking, the recipe for Plant-Based Vegan Stuffed Mushrooms takes about 25 to 30 minutes to prepare.

VEGAN PHO

Ingredients:
For the Broth:

- 1 large onion, halved and unpeeled
- 1 large piece (about 4 inches) of ginger, sliced
- 4-5 cloves garlic, crushed
- 4-5 star anise
- 4-5 whole cloves
- 1 cinnamon stick

- 1 cardamom pod (optional)
- 1 tablespoon coriander seeds
- 1 medium-sized carrot, roughly chopped
- 1-2 tablespoons soy sauce or tamari
- 8 cups vegetable broth
- Salt and sugar to taste

For the Pho Bowl:
- Flat rice noodles, cooked according to package instructions
- Tofu, sliced and pan-fried (optional)
- Bean sprouts
- Fresh basil leaves
- Lime wedges
- Sliced green onions
- Fresh cilantro leaves
- Sriracha sauce (optional)
- Hoisin sauce (optional)

Guidelines:
1. First, grill the onion and ginger: Set your oven's broiler on high. Arrange the ginger slices and onion halves on a baking sheet. They should be broiling for ten to fifteen minutes to get a good char. As an alternative, you can burn them on a gas stove over an open flame.
2. Toast the Spices: - Toast the coriander seeds, cloves, cinnamon stick, star anise, and cardamom pod (if using) on a dry pan until fragrant. Take care not to scorch them.
3. Make the Broth: - Combine the soy sauce or tamari, diced carrot, toasted spices, charred onion,

ginger, smashed garlic, and vegetable broth in a big pot. After bringing to a boil, lower the heat and simmer for 30 to 45 minutes to allow the flavors to fully develop.

4. Strain Broth: Put the clear broth back into the pot after straining out any solids. Add a little sugar and salt to taste.

5. Prepare Toppings: - Assemble the toppings in the midst of cooking the broth. Prepare the rice noodles as directed on the package, sauté the tofu if using it, and reserve the fresh veggies and herbs.

6. Assemble Pho Bowls: - Assemble cooked rice noodles, tofu, bean sprouts, lime wedges, sliced green onions, and cilantro in serving bowls.

7. To serve, top the combined ingredients in each bowl with the heated broth. Serve right away, with Hoisin and Sriracha sauce optionally on the side.

Cooking Time: Including the broth's preparation and simmering, the entire cooking time for Plant-Based Vegan Pho is about 50 to 60 minutes.

QUINOA STUFFED BELL PEPPER

Ingredients:
- 4 large bell peppers, halved and seeds removed
- 1 cup quinoa, rinsed
- 2 cups vegetable broth
- 1 can (15 oz) black beans, drained and rinsed
- 1 cup fresh corn kernels or canned
- 1 cup diced tomatoes
- 1 cup diced red onion

- 1 cup diced zucchini
- 2 cloves garlic, minced
- 1 teaspoon ground cumin
- 1 teaspoon chili powder
- 1/2 teaspoon smoked paprika
- Salt and pepper to taste
- 1 cup tomato sauce
- Vegan shredded cheese for topping (optional)
- Fresh cilantro or parsley for garnish

Guidelines:
1. Preheat Oven: - Set the oven's temperature to 375°F, or 190°C.
2. Prepare the Quinoa: - Put the Quinoa and the veggie broth in a pot. After bringing to a boil, lower the heat to a simmer, cover, and cook the quinoa for 15 to 20 minutes, or until the liquid has been absorbed.
3. Prepare the bell peppers by halves them and taking off the seeds and membranes. Put them inside a dish for baking.
4. Prepare the Filling: - Combine the cooked quinoa, black beans, corn, diced tomatoes, red onion, and zucchini with minced garlic, ground cumin, smoked paprika, chili powder, and salt and pepper in a large bowl. Blend thoroughly.
5. Stuff Bell Peppers: - Spoon the quinoa mixture into each half of the bell pepper, pushing it down a little.
6. Add Sauce on Top: - Drizzle each stuffed pepper with a little tomato sauce. Add some vegan shredded cheese if you'd like.

7. Bake: - Bake the bell peppers in the preheated oven for 25 to 30 minutes, or until they are soft, while covering the baking dish with foil.
8. Garnish and Serve: Take out of the oven, sprinkle with parsley or cilantro, and serve warm.

Cooking Time: Including prep and baking, the Plant-Based Quinoa Stuffed Bell Peppers take about 45 to 50 minutes to make in total.

VEGAN PAD THAI

Ingredients:
- 8 oz rice noodles
- 1 tablespoon vegetable oil
- 1 block (about 14 oz) firm tofu, pressed and cubed
- 1 cup broccoli florets
- 1 carrot, julienned
- 1 bell pepper, thinly sliced
- 2 cloves garlic, minced
- 2 cups bean sprouts
- 3 green onions, sliced
- 1/4 cup peanuts chopped (optional)for garnishing
- Lime wedges for serving

For the Sauce:
- 3 tablespoons soy sauce or tamari
- 2 tablespoons tamarind paste
- 1 tablespoon maple syrup or agave nectar
- 1 tablespoon rice vinegar
- 1 tsp sriracha sauce
- 1 tablespoon vegetable oil

Guidelines:
1. Prepare the rice noodles: - Cook the rice noodles as directed on the package. After draining, set away.
2. Prepare Sauce: - To make the sauce, whisk together soy sauce or tamari, tamarind paste, rice vinegar, sriracha sauce, maple syrup or agave nectar, and vegetable oil in a small bowl. Tailor the tastes to your preference.
3. Cook Tofu: - Heat vegetable oil in a big skillet or wok over medium-high heat. Cook until golden brown on all sides after adding the cubed tofu. Take out the tofu and place it aside.
4. Sauté Vegetables: - If necessary, add a little extra oil to the same pan. Add the broccoli, carrot, bell pepper, and minced garlic and sauté until the veggies are crisp-tender.
5. Mix Tofu and Noodles: - Return the cooked tofu and cooked rice noodles to the pan.
6. Pour Sauce: - Drizzle the noodles and tofu with the prepared sauce. To ensure even coating, combine all ingredients.
7. Add the Bean Sprouts and Green Onions: - Mix in the chopped green onions and the bean sprouts. Simmer for a further two to three minutes, or until the bean sprouts are crisp and slightly cooked.
8. Garnish and Present: - Add chopped peanuts, if desired, to the dish and present it hot with lime wedges on the side.

Cooking Time: Including preparation and cooking, the recipe for Plant-Based Vegan Pad Thai takes about 25 to 30 minutes to complete.

CHICKPEA AND SPINACH STEW

Ingredients:
- 2 tablespoons olive oil
- 1 large onion, finely chopped
- 3 cloves garlic, minced
- 1 teaspoon ground cumin
- 1 teaspoon ground coriander
- 1 teaspoon smoked paprika
- 1/2 teaspoon ground turmeric
- 1/4 tsp cayenne pepper for heat
- 2 cans (15 oz each) chickpeas, washed and rinsed
- 1 can (14 oz) diced tomatoes
- 1 cup vegetable broth
- 1 bay leaf
- Salt and pepper to taste
- 4 cups fresh spinach leaves
- Fresh lemon wedges for serving
- Cooked quinoa or rice for serving (optional)

Guidelines:
1. Sauté Aromatics: - Place a big pot over medium heat with olive oil. Add chopped onion and sauté for 3 to 5 minutes, or until softened.Add minced garlic and sauté for an additional 1-2 minutes.
2. Add Spices: - Add cayenne pepper (if using), smoked paprika, ground cumin, ground coriander,

and ground turmeric. Cook until the spices become fragrant, one to two minutes.

3. Add Tomatoes and Chickpeas: - Fill the saucepan with chopped tomatoes and drained chickpeas. Mix everything together.

4. Add Vegetable Broth: - Add a bay leaf, salt, and pepper to taste, and then pour in the vegetable broth. Simmer the stew for a while.

5. Simmer: To allow the flavors to blend, lower the heat to a simmer, cover the pot, and let the stew cook for 15 to 20 minutes.

6. Add the spinach: - Add the fresh spinach leaves and cook for two to three minutes, or until wilted.

7. Adjust Seasoning: - Taste and make any necessary adjustments to the seasoning. Take out the bay leaf.

8. Present: - Present the heated Chickpea and Spinach Stew, along with freshly cut lemon wedges. Serve over cooked rice or quinoa, if desired.

Cooking Time: Including prep and simmering, the Plant-Based Chickpea and Spinach Stew takes about 25 to 30 minutes to cook in total.

VEGAN SHEPHERD'S PIE

Ingredients:
For the Mashed Potatoes:

- 4 big russet potatoes, peeled and cut into chunks

- 1/2 cup plant-based milk (such as almond, soy, or oat milk)
- 2 tablespoons vegan butter
- Salt and pepper to taste

For the Filling:
- 1 tablespoon olive oil
- 1 large onion, finely chopped
- 2 cloves garlic, minced
- 2 carrots, diced
- 1 cup green peas
- 1 cup corn kernels
- 1 can (15 oz) lentils, drained and rinsed (or cooked green or brown lentils)
- 1 tablespoon tomato paste
- 1 tablespoon soy sauce or tamari
- 1 teaspoon dried thyme
- 1 teaspoon dried rosemary
- 1 cup vegetable broth
- Salt and pepper to taste

Guidelines:
1. To make mashed potatoes, peel and chop the potatoes and put them in a saucepan of salted water. Simmer until potatoes are fork-tender, after bringing to a boil. After draining, mash until smooth with vegan butter, plant-based milk, and salt and pepper. Put aside.
2. Sauté Vegetables: - Heat olive oil in a big skillet over medium heat. Add chopped onion and sauté for 3 to 5 minutes, or until softened. Add the minced garlic and keep on cooking for 1 to 2 minutes.

3. Add Carrots, Peas, and Corn: - Fill the skillet with diced carrots, green peas, and corn. Cook until the vegetables are slightly soft, about 5 more minutes.

4. Prepare Lentil Mixture: - Fill the skillet with the drained lentils, tomato paste, tamari or soy sauce, dried thyme, and dried rosemary. Mix everything together.

5. Add Vegetable Broth: After adding the vegetable broth, boil the mixture for ten to fifteen minutes to enable the flavors to combine. To taste, add salt and pepper for seasoning.

6. Preheat Oven: - Set the oven's temperature to 200°C, or 400°F.

7. Put Shepherd's Pie Together: Place the combination of lentils and vegetables in a baking dish. Evenly distribute the mashed potatoes on top.

8. Bake: - Bake for 20 to 25 minutes, or until the top is golden brown, in a preheated oven.

9. To serve, take it out of the oven and allow it to cool a little. Warm up the food.

Cooking Time: Including prep, cooking, and baking, the Plant-Based Vegan Shepherd's Pie takes about 60 to 70 minutes to prepare.

VEGAN LENTIL LOAF

Ingredients:
For the Lentil Loaf:

- 1 cup dried green or brown lentils, washed and drained

- 2 1/2 cups vegetable broth or you can use water
- 1 tablespoon olive oil
- 1 onion, finely chopped
- 2 carrots, grated
- 2 celery stalks, finely chopped
- 3 cloves garlic, minced
- 1 cup rolled oats
- 1 cup breadcrumbs (ensure they are vegan)
- 1/2 cup tomato sauce or ketchup
- 2 tablespoons soy sauce or tamari
- 1 tablespoon Dijon mustard
- 1 teaspoon dried thyme
- 1 teaspoon dried rosemary
- Salt and pepper to taste

For the Glaze:
- 1/4 cup tomato sauce or ketchup
- 2 tsp maple syrup or agave nectar
- 1 tablespoon balsamic vinegar

Guidelines:
1. Cook Lentils: Put lentils and water or vegetable broth in a pot. After bringing to a boil, lower the heat and simmer the lentils for 25 to 30 minutes, or until they are soft but not mushy. Remove any extra liquid.
2. Sauté Vegetables: - Heat olive oil in a big skillet over medium heat. Add the minced garlic, diced onion, chopped celery, and grated carrots. Sauté the vegetables for five to seven minutes, or until they are tender.

3. Prepare Lentil Mixture: - Mix cooked lentils, sautéed veggies, rolled oats, breadcrumbs, tomato sauce, tamari or soy sauce, Dijon mustard, dried rosemary, dried thyme, and salt and pepper in a big bowl. Toss to blend well.

4. Preheat Oven: - Set the oven's temperature to 375°F, or 190°C.

5. Form the Lentil Loaf: - Spoon the lentil mixture into a loaf pan that has been coated with oil, then flatten it to create a uniform loaf shape.

6. Prepare Glaze: - To make the glaze, whisk together tomato sauce (or ketchup), agave nectar (or maple syrup), and balsamic vinegar in a small basin.

7. Glaze the Loaf: - Evenly cover the top of the lentil loaf with the glaze.

8. Bake: - Bake in the preheated oven for about 40-45 minutes or until the lentil loaf is firm and the top is golden brown.

9. Remain and Present: - Give the lentil loaf a few minutes to settle before slicing. Warm up the food.

Cooking Time: Including prep and baking, the Plant-Based Vegan Lentil Loaf takes about 70 to 75 minutes to cook in total.

VEGAN STUFFED ACORN SQUASH

Ingredients:
- 2 acorn squashes, halved and seeds removed
- 1 cup quinoa, rinsed
- 2 cups vegetable broth

- 1 tablespoon olive oil
- 1 onion, finely chopped
- 2 cloves garlic, minced
- 1 bell pepper, diced
- 1 zucchini, diced
- 1 cup black beans, drained and rinsed
- 1 teaspoon ground cumin
- 1 teaspoon smoked paprika
- Salt and pepper to taste
- 1/2 cup chopped fresh cilantro or parsley
- Juice of 1 lime
- Optional toppings: avocado slices, vegan sour cream, or hot sauce

Guidelines:
1. Get ready the squash: - Turn the oven up to 375°F (190°C). Acorn squash halves should be placed cut-side up on a baking pan. After applying a little olive oil to the sliced sides, season with salt and pepper. Roast the squash for 35 to 40 minutes, or until it is soft to the fork.
2. Prepare Quinoa: In a saucepan, mix quinoa with vegetable broth while the squashes are roasting. After bringing to a boil, lower the heat, cover, and simmer the quinoa for 15 to 20 minutes, or until it is tender and the liquid has been absorbed.
3. Sauté Vegetables: - Heat olive oil in a big skillet over medium heat. Add the diced bell pepper, diced zucchini, minced garlic, and chopped onion. Sauté the vegetables for five to seven minutes, or until they are tender.

4. Mix Quinoa with Vegetables: - Add black beans, smoked paprika, ground cumin, cooked quinoa, salt, and pepper. After thoroughly combining, cook for a further two to three minutes, or until thoroughly cooked.

5. Add Fresh Herbs and Lime Juice: - Turn off the heat and add the chopped parsley or cilantro to the skillet. Add the lime juice to the mixture and stir one last time.

6. insert Squash: After the acorn squashes have finished roasting, insert the vegetable mixture and quinoa into each half.

7. Optional Toppings: - If preferred, place slices of avocado, a dollop of vegan sour cream, or a splash of spicy sauce on top of each stuffed squash.

8. Serve: - Warm up the vegan stuffed acorn squash and savor it.

Cooking Time:- The total cooking time for Plant-Based Vegan Stuffed Acorn Squash is approximately 60-70 minutes, including preparation and roasting.

PLANT-BASED LASAGNA

Ingredients:

For the Lasagna:

- 12 lasagna noodles, cooked according to package instructions
- 1 tablespoon olive oil
- 1 onion, finely chopped
- 3 cloves garlic, minced

- 1 zucchini, diced
- 1 bell pepper, diced
- 1 carrot, grated
- 1 cup mushrooms, sliced
- 1 can (28 oz) crushed tomatoes
- 1 can (15 oz) tomato sauce
- 1 can (6 oz) tomato paste
- 2 teaspoons dried oregano
- 1 teaspoon dried basil
- 1 teaspoon dried thyme
- Salt and pepper to taste

For the Tofu Ricotta:
- 1 block (about 14 oz) firm tofu, drained
- 2 tablespoons nutritional yeast
- 2 tablespoons lemon juice
- 1 teaspoon garlic powder
- Salt and pepper to taste

For Assembly:
- Vegan mozzarella cheese (optional)

Guidelines:
1. Prepare the Vegetables: - Heat the olive oil in a large skillet over medium heat. Add the diced bell pepper, diced zucchini, diced onion, minced garlic, grated carrot, and sliced mushrooms. Sauté the veggies till they get tender.
2. Prepare Tomato Sauce: - Fill the skillet with crushed tomatoes, tomato paste, dried basil, dried thyme, dried oregano, and salt and pepper. Simmer to let the flavors combine, about 15 to 20 minutes.

3. Get the tofu ricotta ready: Drained tofu, nutritional yeast, lemon juice, garlic powder, salt, and pepper should all be combined in a food processor. Process until creamy and smooth, similar to ricotta cheese.

4. Preheat Oven: - Set the oven's temperature to 375°F, or 190°C.

5. Put the lasagna together: - Cover the bottom of a baking dish with tomato sauce. Cover with a layer of cooked lasagna noodles. Start with a layer of tofu ricotta, then top with a layer of tomato sauce and, if you'd like, some vegan mozzarella cheese. Continue layering ingredients until all are utilized, and then top with a layer of tomato sauce.

6. Bake: - Bake the baking dish for around 30 to 35 minutes in a preheated oven, covered with foil. For the final ten minutes, take off the foil to let the top softly brown.

7. Rest and Serve: - Before slicing, let the lasagna sit for a few minutes. Warm up the food.

Cooking Time:- The total cooking time for Plant-Based Lasagna is approximately 60-70 minutes, including preparation and baking.

CHICKPEA STIR-FRY WITH BROCCOLI

Ingredients:
- 1 can (15 oz) chickpeas, drained and rinsed
- 2 tablespoons soy sauce or tamari

- 1 tablespoon rice vinegar
- 1 tsp maple syrup or agave nectar
- 1 tablespoon sesame oil
- 1 tablespoon cornstarch
- 1 tablespoon vegetable oil
- 3 cups broccoli florets
- 1 bell pepper, thinly sliced
- 1 carrot, julienned
- 3 cloves garlic, minced
- 1 tablespoon fresh ginger, grated
- Cooked brown rice or quinoa for serving
- For garnishing sesame seeds and green onions

Guidelines:

1. Let the chickpeas marinate: Chickpeas, rice vinegar, agave nectar or maple syrup, cornstarch, sesame oil, and soy sauce or tamari should all be combined in a bowl. Give the chickpeas ten to fifteen minutes to marinade.

2. Sauté the chickpeas: - Heat the vegetable oil in a big skillet or wok over medium-high heat. When the chickpeas are golden brown and beginning to crisp up, add the marinated ones and simmer. Take out and place aside the chickpeas from the skillet.

3. Vegetable Stir-Fry: - If necessary, add a little extra oil to the same skillet. When the vegetables are soft and crisp, sauté broccoli, bell pepper, julienned carrot, minced garlic, and grated ginger.

4. Combine Vegetables and Chickpeas: - Return the cooked chickpeas to the skillet along with the stir-fried veggies. Mix everything together until thoroughly hot and properly mixed.

5. Serve: - Top cooked brown rice or quinoa with the chickpea stir-fry. Add sliced green onions and sesame seeds as garnish.

Cooking Time: Including marinating and stir-frying, the Plant-Based Chickpea Stir-Fry with Broccoli takes about 30 to 35 minutes to cook in total.

VEGAN LENTIL TACOS

Ingredients:
For the Lentil Filling:
- 1 cup dry green or brown lentils, rinsed
- 3 cups vegetable broth
- 1 tablespoon olive oil
- 1 onion, finely chopped
- 2 cloves garlic, minced
- 1 can (15 oz) diced tomatoes
- 1 tablespoon tomato paste
- 1 tablespoon chili powder
- 1 teaspoon ground cumin
- 1 teaspoon paprika
- 1/2 teaspoon dried oregano
- Salt and pepper to taste

For Taco Assembly:
- Corn or flour tortillas
- Shredded lettuce
- Diced tomatoes
- Sliced avocado
- Salsa
- Vegan sour cream

- Fresh cilantro, chopped
- Lime wedges

Guidelines:
1. Cook Lentils: - Place rinsed lentils and vegetable broth in a saucepan. Once the lentils are soft, reduce the heat and simmer for 20 to 25 minutes after bringing to a boil. Remove any extra liquid.
2. Sauté the onion and garlic: - Heat the olive oil in a big skillet over medium heat. When the onion is soft, add it diced and sauté it. Add the minced garlic and keep to cooking for 1 to 2 minutes.
3. Add Lentils and Spices: - Include diced tomatoes, tomato paste, ground cumin, paprika, dried oregano, chili powder, and salt and pepper in the skillet with the cooked lentils. After thoroughly mixing, simmer for a further ten to fifteen minutes to let the flavors blend.
4. Prepare Taco Toppings: - While the lentil filling is simmering, chop the cilantro, slice the avocado, shred the lettuce, and dice the tomatoes.
5. Warm Tortillas: - Follow the directions on the package to reheat the tortillas on a dry skillet or the microwave.
6. Assemble Tacos: - Transfer each tortilla with a spoonful of lentil filling. Add chopped cilantro, salsa, vegan sour cream, diced tomatoes, sliced avocado, and shredded lettuce on top.
7. Present: - Accompany the Vegan Lentil Tacos with wedges of lime.

Cooking Time: Including preparation and simmering, the Plant-Based Vegan Lentil Tacos take about 40 to 45 minutes to make in total.

VEGAN RATATOUILLE

Ingredients:
- 1 large eggplant, sliced into rounds
- 2 medium zucchinis, sliced into rounds
- 1 large bell pepper, thinly sliced
- 1 large red onion, thinly sliced
- 3 medium tomatoes, sliced into rounds
- 4 cloves garlic, minced
- 2 tablespoons tomato paste
- 2 tablespoons olive oil
- 1 teaspoon dried thyme
- 1 teaspoon dried rosemary
- 1 teaspoon dried oregano
- Salt and pepper to taste
- Fresh basil for garnish

Guidelines:
1. Get the vegetables ready. - Turn the oven on to 375°F (190°C). Cut the bell pepper, tomatoes, zucchini, eggplant, and red onion into rounds.
2. Layer Vegetables: - Place the sliced eggplant, zucchini, bell pepper, red onion, and tomato in an overlapping manner in a baking dish. Until the dish is full, keep going.
3. Prepare the Tomato Sauce: - Combine the tomato paste, olive oil, dried oregano, dried thyme,

dried rosemary, and salt and pepper in a small bowl. Drizzle this mixture onto the veggie layers.
4. Bake: - Bake the baking dish for 45 to 50 minutes in a preheated oven, covered with foil. After uncovered, bake the veggies for a further 15 to 20 minutes, or until they are soft and beginning to brown.
5. Garnish and Serve: Take out of the oven, top with freshly chopped basil, and serve warm.

Cooking Time: Including preparation and baking, the Vegan Ratatouille takes about 60 to 70 minutes to cook in total.

MUSHROOM RISOTTO

Ingredients:
- 1 1/2 cups Arborio rice
- 1/2 cup dry white wine
- 5 cups vegetable broth, kept warm
- 1 tablespoon olive oil
- 1 medium onion, finely chopped
- 2 cloves garlic, minced
- 8 oz (about 225g) mushrooms (such as cremini or shiitake), sliced
- 1 cup fresh spinach, chopped
- 1/2 cup nutritional yeast
- 1 tablespoon vegan butter
- Salt and black pepper to taste
- Fresh parsley for garnish (optional)

Guidelines:
1. Sauté the Mushrooms: - Heat the olive oil in a big skillet or saucepan over medium heat. When the onion is soft, add it diced and sauté it. Add the chopped garlic and the sliced mushrooms, and cook them until they turn golden brown.
2. Toast Rice: - Place the Arborio rice in the skillet and toss to coat it with oil, cooking it for one to two minutes.
3. Use Wine to Deglaze: - Add the dry white wine and stir until the majority of the liquid evaporates.
4. Add Broth: - Stir frequently as you add one ladle at a time of the heated vegetable broth. Don't add the next ladle until the majority of the liquid has been absorbed. Once the rice is creamy and cooked to your preference, keep on with this process. Usually, this takes between 18 and 20 minutes.
5. Stir in Spinach and Nutritional Yeast: - Add the chopped spinach about halfway through the cooking time. Add more broth until the rice is cooked through. Add nutritional yeast and stir.
6. Add Vegan Butter to Finish: - After the risotto is cooked, whisk in vegan butter. To taste, add salt and black pepper for seasoning.
7. Garnish and Serve: - If preferred, sprinkle fresh parsley over the mushroom risotto. Warm up the food.

Cooking Time: - Preparation and cooking of the plant-based mushroom risotto take about 25 to 30 minutes in total.

VEGAN BURRITO BOWL

Ingredients:

For the Burrito Bowl
- 1 cup quinoa or brown rice cooked
- 1 can (15 oz) black beans,washed and rinsed
- 1 cup corn kernels (fresh,or canned)
- 1 cup cherry tomatoes, halved
- 1 avocado, sliced
- 1 cup shredded lettuce or kale
- 1/2 cup red onion, finely chopped
- Fresh cilantro for garnish

For the Lime Cilantro Dressing:
- 1/4 cup fresh lime juice
- 2 tablespoons olive oil
- 2 tablespoons chopped fresh cilantro
- 1 teaspoon maple syrup or agave nectar
- Salt and pepper to taste

Guidelines:

1. Prepare the quinoa or brown rice: Follow the directions on the package to cook the quinoa or brown rice.
2. Assemble Burrito Bowls: - Arrange cooked quinoa or brown rice, chopped red onion, black beans, corn kernels, avocado slices, cherry tomatoes, shredded lettuce or kale, and diced avocado in serving bowls.
3. Prepare the Lime-Cilantro Dressing: To make the dressing, combine the olive oil, chopped cilantro,

maple syrup or agave nectar, fresh lime juice, salt, and pepper in a small bowl.
4. Drizzle Dressing: - Cover the burrito bowl with a drizzle of the lime cilantro dressing.
Garnish and Serve: - Sprinkle freshly chopped cilantro on top and serve right away.

Cooking Time: Including preparation and assembly, a vegan burrito bowl takes about 20 to 25 minutes to prepare in total.

CHAPTER FIVE

DELICIOUS DESSERTS

ALMOND BUTTER ENERGY BALLS

Ingredients:
- 1 cup rolled oats
- 1/2 cup almond butter
- 1/3 cup maple syrup or agave nectar
- 1/2 cup ground flaxseed
- 1 teaspoon vanilla extract
- A pinch of salt
- Optional: 1/3 cup chopped nuts, seeds, or shredded coconut for coating

Guidelines
1. Place rolled oats, almond butter, maple syrup, ground flaxseed, vanilla essence, and a small amount of salt in a big bowl.
2. Fully combine the ingredients by mixing them together. You can add extra oats or briefly chill the mixture if it's too sticky.
3. To make the mixture simpler to handle, chill it for 15 to 30 minutes after it has been thoroughly mixed.
4. Once the mixture has cooled, divide it into little sections and shape them into bite-sized balls. For

added taste and texture, you can optionally roll the balls with chopped nuts, seeds, or shredded coconut.

5. To firm up, place the energy balls on a dish coated with parchment paper and refrigerate for a minimum of 30 more minutes.

6. After the energy balls are hard, place them in an airtight container and refrigerate.

MATCHA GREEN TEA ICE CREAM

Ingredients:
- 2 cans (28 oz) full-fat coconut milk, chilled
- 1/2 cup agave nectar or maple syrup
- 2 tablespoons matcha green tea powder
- 1 teaspoon vanilla extract

Guidelines
1. Make sure the coconut milk cans are thoroughly refrigerated in the fridge for a minimum of six hours or overnight.

2. Without shaking them, open the cans of cold coconut milk. Remove the thick coconut cream from the top and transfer it to a bowl, discarding the liquid (you may use it in smoothies or other recipes).

3. Put the matcha green tea powder, coconut cream, vanilla extract, and agave nectar (or maple syrup) in a blender.

4. Puree the blend until it's creamy and smooth.

5. Transfer the mixture to an ice cream machine and process it in accordance with the

manufacturer's directions until it thickens to the consistency of soft serve.

6. Spoon the ice cream into a container with a cover, level the top, and freeze for a minimum of 4 hours, or until solid.

VEGAN CHOCOLATE AVOCADO COOKIES

Ingredients:
- 1 ripe avocado, mashed
- 1/2 cup coconut sugar or other sweetener
- 1/4 cup cocoa powder
- 1 cup oat flour (blend oats to make flour)
- 1/2 teaspoon baking powder
- 1/4 teaspoon salt
- 1/2 cup dairy-free chocolate chips or chopped dark chocolate
- 1 teaspoon vanilla extract

Guidelines:
1. Preheat the oven to 350°F (175°C) and place parchment paper on a baking pan.
2. Thoroughly mix the mashed avocado and coconut sugar in a bowl.
3. Include chocolate chips, vanilla extract, baking powder, oat flour, cocoa powder, and salt in the avocado mixture. Stir to form a dough.
4. Leaving space between each cookie, scoop spoonfuls of dough onto the baking sheet that has been prepared.

5. Since these cookies won't spread much as they bake, gently press each one down with the back of a spoon or your fingertips.
6. Bake for 10 to 12 minutes, or until the edges are firm, in a preheated oven.
7. Let the cookies cool for a few minutes on the baking sheet, then move them to a wire rack to finish cooling.

VEGAN TIRAMISU

Ingredients
For the Soaking Liquid Coffee:
- One cup of strongly brewed, chilled coffee
- 2 tablespoons of agave nectar or maple syrup
 - 1 tablespoon of optional coffee liqueur

To make the Cashew Cream:
 - 1/2 cup coconut milk
- 1 1/2 cups raw cashews soaked in water for at least 4 hours or overnight
- 1/4 cup melted coconut oil
 - 1/2 cup maple syrup or agave nectar
 - 1 teaspoon vanilla essence - A pinch of salt
Extra Ingredients:
- Enough vegan ladyfinger cookies to cover the bottom of the dish
Powdered cocoa for dusting

Guidelines:

1. To make the soaking liquid, combine the brewed coffee, agave nectar or maple syrup, and coffee liqueur (if using) in a shallow dish.
2. Put the cashews that have been soaked, coconut milk, melted coconut oil, vanilla extract, maple syrup or agave nectar, and a dash of salt in a blender. Blend till creamy and smooth.
3. Make sure the vegan ladyfingers are moist but not too wet by dipping them into the coffee soaking liquid. Line the bottom of your serving plate with a layer of moistened ladyfingers.
4. Cover the layer of ladyfingers with half of the cashew cream.
5. Repeat with the remaining cashew cream and another layer of soaked ladyfingers.
6. Sprinkle chocolate powder over top.
7. To let the flavors combine, place the tiramisu in the refrigerator for at least four hours or overnight.

VEGAN CHOCOLATE CAKE

Ingredients:
For the Cake:
- 2 cups all-purpose flour
- 1 1/2 cups granulated sugar
- 3/4 cup cocoa powder
- 1 1/2 teaspoons baking powder
- 1 1/2 teaspoons baking soda
- 1 teaspoon salt
- 1 1/2 cups soy milk or almond milk non-dairy
- 1/2 cup vegetable oil
- 2 teaspoons vanilla extract

- 1 cup hot water or brewed coffee

For the Frosting:
- 1/2 cup vegan butter, softened
- 2/3 cup cocoa powder
- 3 cups powdered sugar
- 1/3 cup non-dairy milk
- 1 teaspoon vanilla extract

Guidelines:
1. Grease two 9-inch round cake pans and preheat the oven to 350°F (175°C).
2. Combine the flour, sugar, baking soda, baking powder, cocoa powder, and salt in a sizable mixing basin.
3. Combine the dry ingredients with the non dairy milk, vegetable oil, and vanilla essence. Blend until thoroughly blended.
4. Add the hot water or coffee and stir until the batter is well combined. There will be a thin batter; this is expected.
5. Evenly divide the batter among the cake pans that have been prepared, then smooth the tops.
6. Bake for 30 to 35 minutes, or until a toothpick inserted in the center comes out clean, in a preheated oven.
7. After letting the cakes cool in the pans for ten minutes, move them to a wire rack to finish cooling.
8. To make the frosting, blend vegan butter, powdered sugar, cocoa powder, non-dairy milk, and vanilla extract until they become smooth and creamy.

9. After the cakes are fully cool, frost one cake layer's top, then top that layer with the second layer and cover the whole cake with frosting.

CHOCOLATE AVOCADO PUDDING

Ingredients:
- 1/2 cup cocoa powder - 2 ripe avocados, pitted and peeled
- 1/2 cup of agave nectar or maple syrup
- 1/2 cup of plant-based milk (almond or coconut)
- One tsp vanilla essence
- A dash of salt

Instructions:
1. Place the ripe avocados, cocoa powder, plant-based milk, vanilla extract, maple syrup or agave nectar, and a dash of salt in a blender or food processor.
2. Puree the mixture until it's creamy and smooth. To make sure everything is thoroughly combined, you might need to pause and scrape down the sides of the food processor or blender.
3. After tasting the pudding, modify its thickness or sweetness by adding more plant-based milk or sweetener as necessary.
4. Spoon the pudding into glasses or serving dishes after it has reached a smooth consistency.
5. To enable the chocolate avocado pudding to chill and firm slightly, place it in the refrigerator for at least 30 minutes before serving.

VEGAN APPLE CRISP

Ingredients:

The Filling:

Six cups of peeled and sliced apples (preferably Granny Smith or Honeycrisp) - One tablespoon of lemon juice - 1/4 cup of maple syrup or agave nectar

- One teaspoon of ground cinnamon
- 1/4 teaspoon of nutmeg, ground

The Topping:

One cup of old-fashioned oats, half a cup of all-purpose flour, and half a cup of chopped nuts (almonds or walnuts)

One-fourth cup brown sugar or coconut sugar

- 1/4 cup vegan butter or melted coconut oil
- One teaspoon of ground cinnamon
- A scant teaspoon of salt

Guidelines:

Adjust the oven temperature to 350°F (175°C) and coat a baking dish with oil.

2. Put the apple slices, agave nectar or maple syrup, lemon juice, grated nutmeg, and cinnamon in a big bowl. Until the apples are evenly covered, toss.

3. Evenly lay out the apple mixture in the baking dish that has been prepared.

4. Combine the oats, flour, chopped nuts, melted coconut oil or vegan butter, ground cinnamon, and

a small amount of salt in another bowl. Mix the mixture until it becomes crumbly.

5. Evenly distribute the oat topping over the baking dish's apple mixture.

6. Bake for 40 to 45 minutes in a preheated oven, or until the apples are soft and the topping is golden brown.

7. Before serving, let the vegan apple crisp cool a little.

NO-BAKE VEGAN CHEESECAKE BITES

Ingredients:

For the Crust:
- 1 cup dates, pitted
- 1 cup of almonds or cashews nuts
- A pinch of salt

For the Cheesecake Filling:
- 2 cups raw cashew nuts soaked in water for 4 hours at least or overnight
- 1/2 cup coconut cream
- 1/3 cup maple syrup or agave nectar
- 1/4 cup coconut oil, melted
- 1 teaspoon vanilla extract
- Juice of 1 lemon

For the Topping:
- Fresh berries or fruit of your

Guidelines:

1. To make the crust, pulse nuts, pitted dates, and a small teaspoon of salt in a food processor. Process until the mixture holds together and becomes sticky.

2. To form the base of the cheesecake bites, press the crust mixture firmly onto the bottom of a square baking sheet or a prepared mini-muffin tin.

3. Put the soaked cashews, coconut cream, agave nectar or maple syrup, melted coconut oil, vanilla extract, and lemon juice in a blender. Blend till creamy and smooth.

4. Using a spatula to smooth the tops, spoon the cheesecake filling over the crust in the muffin tray or baking pan.

5. Put the cheesecake bits in the freezer to solidify for a minimum of four hours.

6. After the cheesecake bites are set, take them out of the freezer and allow them to come to room temperature for a couple of minutes before taking them out of the muffin tray.

7. Add your choice of fruit, or fresh berries, on the top of each cheesecake bite.

COCONUT MANGO SORBET

Ingredients:
- 2 ripe mangoes, peeled and diced
- 1 can (14 oz) chilled coconut milk
- 1/2 cup agave nectar or maple syrup
- 1 tablespoon lime juice
- A pinch of salt

Directions:

1. Put the chopped mangoes in a food processor or blender and mix until smooth.
2. Combine cooled coconut milk, lime juice, agave nectar or maple syrup, and a dash of salt in another bowl.
3. Blend the coconut milk mixture thoroughly after adding the mango puree.
4. Fill a shallow dish with the sorbet mixture, cover it, and freeze.
5. Use a fork to stir the sorbet every 30 minutes to break up any ice crystals. Continue doing this for three to four hours, or until the sorbet has the consistency of a smooth, scoopable gel.
6. Spoon the sorbet into bowls or cones and serve as soon as it sets.

VEGAN BANANA BREAD

Ingredients:

- 3 ripe bananas, mashed
- 1/3 cup coconut oil or vegetable oil melted
- 1/2 cup maple or agave syrup
- 1 teaspoon vanilla extract
- 1 teaspoon baking soda
- A pinch of salt
- 1 3/4 cups all-purpose flour or whole wheat flour
- 1/4 cup plant-based milk (such as almond or soy)
- 1 teaspoon apple cider vinegar (to react with baking soda)

Guidelines:

1. Grease a 9 by 5-inch loaf pan and preheat the oven to 350°F (175°C).
2. Using a fork or potato masher, mash the ripe bananas in a large mixing dish.
3. Mix the mashed bananas with vanilla essence, heated coconut oil or vegetable oil, and maple syrup or agave nectar. Blend thoroughly.
4. Mix the plant-based milk and apple cider vinegar in a different small bowl. Give it time to curdle, a few minutes at most.
5. Stir the banana mixture thoroughly after adding the curdled milk.
6. Sift the flour, baking soda, and a little amount of salt into the same basin. Do not overmix; just blend the ingredients.
7. Transfer the mixture into the loaf pan that has been ready and level the top.
8. Bake for 60 to 70 minutes, or until a toothpick inserted in the center comes out clean, in a preheated oven.
9. After letting the vegan banana bread cool in the pan for ten or so minutes, move it to a wire rack to finish cooling.

PISTACHIO DATES BITES

Ingredients:
- 1 cup pitted dates
- 1/2 cup shelled pistachios
- 1/4 cup unsweetened shredded coconut
- 1 tablespoon chia seeds

- 1 tablespoon almond butter or any nut/seed butter of your choice
- A pinch of salt

Guidelines
1. Place the almond butter, shredded coconut, chia seeds, pitted dates, shelled pistachios, and a dash of salt in a food processor.
2. Mix the ingredients until a sticky dough forms. With your fingertips, you should be able to press it together.
3. Using your hands, scoop out tiny parts of the dough and shape them into bite-sized balls.
4. Optional: Coat the balls with finely chopped pistachios or more shredded coconut.
5. Transfer the bite-sized pistachio dates to a parchment paper-lined platter or tray.
6. To firm up, refrigerate the bits for a minimum of half an hour.

VEGAN CINNAMON ROLLS

Ingredients:
For the Dough:
- 1 cup non-dairy milk (such as almond or soy), warmed
- 1 packet 2 1/4 tablespoon active dry yeast
- 1/4 cup granulated sugar
- 1/3 cup vegan butter, melted
- 3 1/2 cups all-purpose flour
- 1/2 teaspoon salt
For the Filling:

- 1/2 cup vegan butter, softened
- 3/4 cup brown sugar, packed
- 2 tablespoons ground cinnamon

For the Icing:
- 1 cup powdered sugar
- 1-2 tablespoons non-dairy milk
- 1/2 teaspoon vanilla extract

Guidelines:
1. Place the granulated sugar, active dry yeast, and warmed nondairy milk in a small bowl. Leave it sit for 5 minutes until foamy
2. Combine the flour, salt, and melted vegan butter in a sizable mixing bowl. When a soft dough forms, add the yeast mixture and continue to combine.
3. Using a floured surface, knead the dough for approximately five minutes, or until it becomes smooth. After putting it in a greased bowl and covering it with a fresh kitchen towel, let it rise in a warm location for one to one and a half hours, or until doubled in size.
4. Oil a baking dish and preheat your oven to 375°F (190°C).
On a surface dusted with flour, roll out the dough to a large rectangle.
6. Cover the rolled-out dough with the softened vegan butter. Combine the ground cinnamon and brown sugar, then evenly distribute it over the butter.

7. To create a log, tightly roll the dough starting from one of the longer sides. Slice the log into rolls of the same size.

8. After the rolls are in the baking dish that has been oiled, give them another 15 to 20 minutes to rise.

9. Bake the rolls for 20 to 25 minutes, or until they are golden brown, in a preheated oven.

10. Make the icing by combining powdered sugar, non-dairy milk, and vanilla essence while the rolls bake.

11. While the rolls are still warm, pour the icing over them right after taking them out of the oven.

RASPBERRY ALMOND THUMBPRINT COOKIES

Ingredients:
For the Cookies:
- 1 cup almond flour
- 1 cup oats rolled gluten-free if need be.
- 1/4 cup coconut oil, melted
- 1/4 cup maple or agave syrup
- 1 teaspoon almond extract
- A pinch of salt

For the Raspberry Filling:
- 1/2 cup raspberry jam or preserves (preferably fruit-sweetened)

Guidelines:

1. Preheat the oven to 350°F (175°C) and place parchment paper on a baking pan.
2. Process almond flour, rolled oats, melted coconut oil, agave nectar or maple syrup, almond extract, and a small amount of salt in a food processor until a dough forms.
3. Using a spoon, scoop out tiny bits of dough and shape them into balls. After the baking sheet is ready, place the balls on it.
4. Make an indentation in the middle of each cookie with your thumb or the back of a spoon.
5. Using approximately 1/2 teaspoon of raspberry jam for each cookie, fill each indentation.
6. Bake for 10 to 12 minutes, or until the cookies' edges are golden brown, in a preheated oven.
7. Let the cookies cool for a few minutes on the baking sheet, then move them to a wire rack to finish cooling.

STRAWBERRY BANANA NICE CREAM

Ingredients:
- 2 ripe bananas, sliced and frozen
- 1 cup frozen strawberries
- 1/4 cup plant-based milk (such as almond or coconut)
- 1 teaspoon vanilla extract (optional)

Instructions:
1. Fill a blender or food processor with the frozen banana slices and frozen strawberries.

2. Include the vanilla essence (if using) and plant-based milk.

3. Process the mixture until it's creamy and smooth. To guarantee even mixing, you might need to stop and scrape down the sides.

4. You can add a little extra plant-based milk to the excellent cream if it's too thick to get the right consistency.

5. Spoon the lovely cream into cones or bowls when it has been combined.

6. Optional: Add more sliced strawberries or your other preferred toppings on top.

7. Present right away and savor your delectable plant-based Banana Nice Cream with Strawberry

CHOCOLATE DIPPED STRAWBERRIES

Ingredients:

- 1 cup dairy
- Fresh strawberries that have been cleaned and dried-free chopped or chips made of dark chocolate
- One tablespoon of coconut oil
- Optional coating ingredients: chopped almonds, shredded coconut, or sprinkles

Guidelines:

1. Use parchment paper to line a tray or dish.

2. Combine the dairy-free dark chocolate and coconut oil in a heatproof basin and melt them together. This can be accomplished with a double boiler or by microwaving in brief bursts of 20 to 30

seconds, stirring in between until the mixture melts completely.

3. Using the stem as a support, immerse each strawberry into the melted chocolate, swirling to coat it completely.

4. Gently shake the strawberries or let any extra chocolate fall off.

5. Optional: For extra taste and flair, roll the chocolate-covered strawberry in chopped almonds, crushed coconut, or sprinkles.

6. Transfer the dipped strawberries to the plate or tray that has been ready.

7. Permit the chocolate to solidify. You can expedite this procedure by chilling the tray for a duration of 15 to 20 minutes.

8. Your plant-based Chocolate Dipped Strawberries are ready to eat once the chocolate has set completely

AVOCADO CHOCOLATE MOUSSE

Ingredients:
- 2 ripe avocados, peeled and pitted
- 1/4 cup cocoa powder
- 1/4 cup maple syrup or agave nectar
- 1/4 cup plant-based milk (such as almond or coconut)
- 1 teaspoon vanilla extract
- A pinch of salt

Instructions:

1. Place the ripe avocados, cocoa powder, plant-based milk, vanilla extract, maple syrup or agave nectar, and a dash of salt in a blender or food processor.
2. Puree the mixture until it's creamy and smooth. To make sure everything is thoroughly combined, you might need to pause and scrape down the sides.
3. After tasting the mousse, add more sweetener or plant-based milk if necessary to change the thickness or sweetness.
4. Spoon the mousse into glasses or serving bowls after it has reached a smooth consistency.
5. To allow the avocado chocolate mousse to cool and firm slightly, place it in the refrigerator for at least 30 minutes before serving.
6. As an optional garnish, you can add some chopped nuts, fresh berries, or a dollop of dairy-free whipped cream before serving.

VEGAN BLUEBERRY CHEESECAKES

Ingredients:
For the Crust:
- 1 1/2 cups graham cracker crumbs (check for vegan options)
- 1/3 cup melted vegan butter
- 2 tablespoons maple syrup

For the Cheesecake Filling:
- 2 cups raw cashew nuts soaked in water for about 4 hours or overnight

- 1/2 cup coconut cream
- 1/2 cup maple or agave syrup
- 1/4 cup melted coconut oil
- 1/4 cup lemon juice
- 1 teaspoon vanilla extract
- A pinch of salt

For the Blueberry Topping:
- 2 cups fresh or frozen blueberries
- 1/4 cup maple or agave syrup
- 1 tablespoon lemon juice
- 1 tablespoon water
- 1 tablespoon cornstarch (optional, for thickening)

Guidelines:
1. Line the bottom of a springform cake pan with parchment paper and preheat the oven to 350°F (175°C).
2. To make the crust, combine the graham cracker crumbs, maple syrup, and melted vegan butter in a bowl. Fill the prepared pan to the brim with the ingredients.
3. Put the soaked cashews, coconut cream, melted coconut oil, lemon juice, vanilla extract, agave nectar, and a dash of salt in a blender. Blend till creamy and smooth.
4. Cover the pan's crust with the cheesecake filling, smoothing the top.
5. Bake for 40 to 45 minutes, or until the middle is still slightly jiggly, in a preheated oven.

6. After letting the cheesecake cool to room temperature, place it in the refrigerator to set for at least four hours or overnight.
7. Put the blueberries, water, lemon juice, and either maple syrup or agave nectar in a saucepan. Mix in some cornstarch that has been dissolved in a little water for a thicker topping.
8. Cook, stirring regularly, the blueberry mixture over medium heat until it thickens. Give it time to cool.
9. Cover the cheesecake's surface with the blueberry topping after it has set.
10. Before serving, refrigerate the cheesecake one more for at least one to two hours.

VEGAN LEMON BARS

Ingredients:
For the Crust:
- 1 cup all-purpose flour
- 1/2 cup vegan butter, softened
- 1/4 cup powdered sugar

For the Lemon Filling:
- 1 1/2 cups granulated sugar
- 1/4 cup cornstarch
- 1/2 teaspoon baking powder
- 1/4 teaspoon turmeric (for color)
- 1/2 cup lemon juice (about 3-4 lemons)
- Zest of 1 lemon
- 1/2 cup plant-based soya or almond milk
Additional Powdered Sugar for Dusting

Guidelines:

Preheat the oven to 350°F (175°C), and place parchment paper inside an 8-by-8-inch baking pan.

2. To make the crust, combine the flour, powdered sugar, and softened vegan butter in a bowl. Stir until crumbly.

3. Evenly press the crust mixture into the pan that has been prepared.

4. Bake the crust for 15 to 18 minutes, or until it is just beginning to turn brown, in a preheated oven.

5. Make the lemon filling while the crust bakes. Combine sugar, cornstarch, baking powder, turmeric, lemon juice, lemon zest, and plant-based milk in a bowl and whisk until thoroughly blended.

6. After the crust has finished baking, pour the lemon filling over it.

7. Put the pan back in the oven and continue to bake for another 20 to 25 minutes, or until the edges

8. Let the lemon bars in the pan cool fully. After cooling, place in the refrigerator to set for at least two hours.

9. After the lemon bars are cold, pull the parchment paper and take them out of the pan onto a chopping board.

10. Cut into squares after dusting the top with powdered sugar.

PEANUT BUTTER OAT COOKIES

Ingredients:

- One cup of rolled oats, without gluten if necessary
- Half a cup of smooth peanut butter
1/4 cup agave nectar or maple syrup
 - 1 mashed ripe banana
- Half a teaspoon of essence from vanilla
- A scant teaspoon of salt
- Optional: 1/2 cup chopped almonds or vegan chocolate chips

Guidelines:
1. Preheat the oven to 350°F (175°C) and place parchment paper on a baking pan.
2. Place the mashed banana, vanilla essence, rolled oats, creamy peanut butter, maple syrup or agave nectar, and a dash of salt in a large mixing basin.
3. Thoroughly blend the ingredients together. Add chopped nuts or vegan chocolate chips, if preferred.
4. Using a spoon, scoop out pieces of dough and place them, spacing them apart, on the baking sheet that has been prepared.
5. Using your fingers or the back of a spoon, slightly flatten each cookie.
6. Bake for 10 to 12 minutes, or until the edges are golden brown, in a preheated oven.
7. Let the cookies cool for a few minutes on the baking sheet before moving them to a wire rack to cool off completely

PUMPKIN SPICE ENERGY BITES

Ingredients:
- 1 cup rolled oats
- 1/2 cup canned pumpkin puree
- 1/4 cup almond butter or any nut/seed butter of your choice
- 1/4 cup maple or agave syrup
- 1 teaspoon pumpkin spice mix (or a combination of cinnamon, nutmeg, ginger, and cloves)
- 1/2 teaspoon vanilla extract
- A pinch of salt
- Optional: Chopped nuts, seeds, or shredded coconut for coating

Guidelines:
Rolled oats, canned pumpkin puree, almond butter, maple syrup or agave nectar, pumpkin spice blend, vanilla essence, and a dash of salt should all be combined in a big mixing bowl.
2. Thoroughly combine the ingredients by mixing them. For extra texture, feel free to fold in chopped nuts, seeds, or shredded coconut.
3. To slightly firm up the mixture, refrigerate it for 15 to 30 minutes.
4. After the mixture has cooled, divide it into small sections and use your hands to roll them into bite-sized balls.
5. Optional: Coat the energy bits with shredded coconut, chopped almonds, or seeds.
6. Arrange the energy bits on a parchment paper-lined dish or tray.

7. Before serving, place the energy bites in the refrigerator for at least half an hour.

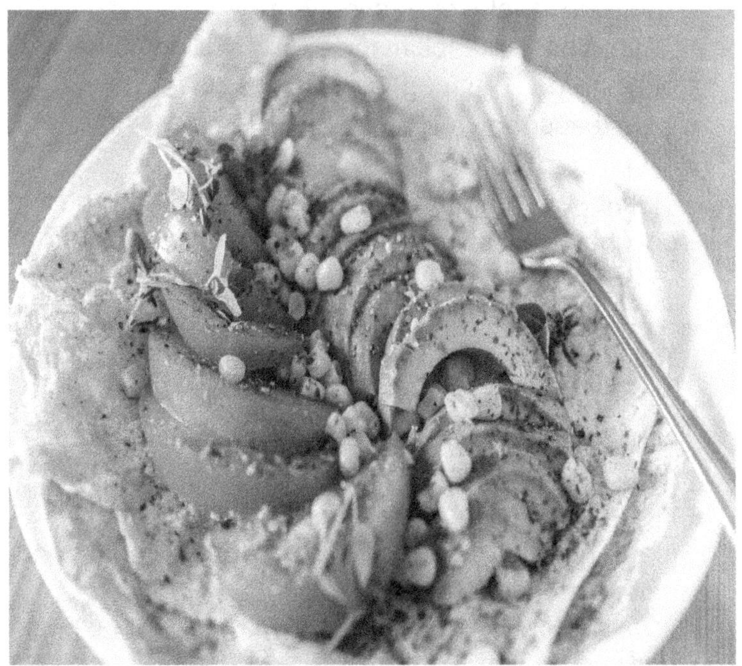

Conclusion

As a culinary compass, The Plant-Based Cookbook for Beginners 2024 points people in the direction of a healthier and more sustainable way of living. At the end of this culinary adventure, we find not just a compilation of recipes but also evidence of the increasing understanding and admiration for plant-based lifestyles.

By the time you turn the last pages of this cookbook, you'll see that adopting a plant-based diet is a transforming choice for your lifestyle rather than just a fad. The recipes in these pages are a celebration of nature's brilliant colors, textures, and flavors, not just a means of subsistence. After reading this gastronomic investigation, readers will have a deeper comprehension of the significant influence that food choices may have on one's own health as well as the environment

In a world where people are becoming more aware of their environmental impact, this cookbook offers a ray of hope. It persuasively shows that leading a plant-based lifestyle is not only doable but also wonderfully tasty. The end of the book signifies not just the end of a book but also the start of a culinary revolution, inspiring readers to learn the skill of plant-based cuisine and set out on a path of self-discovery.

This cookbook's appeal stems not only from its recipes but also from its capacity to help novices understand plant-based cooking. The closing remarks resound with a feeling of empowerment, reassuring readers that they have the abilities and know-how to successfully negotiate this new culinary terrain. It instills trust in the kitchen and eliminates any residual uncertainties regarding the viability of adopting a plant-based lifestyle.

www.ingramcontent.com/pod-product-compliance
Lightning Source LLC
Chambersburg PA
CBHW070847260726
48661CB00004B/1284